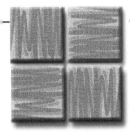

# Foreword

Internet innovations are fueling an exponential increase in the use of the Internet by both health professionals and the public seeking responsible information regarding complementary, alternative, and integrative medicine. As interactive systems, personalized assessments, and international access to products and services increase, there is an equally bewildering array of fragmented, contradictory, and often unfounded recommendations and claims. What is needed is an "evidence-based" or research outcomes approach that will allow both health professionals and the public to make truly informed decisions regarding their personal health care and that of their family.

With this innovative book, Mac Beckner and Brian Berman, M.D., of the Complementary Medicine Program (CMP) at the University of Maryland School of Medicine have achieved that objective with a thoughtful, accessible, evidence-based guide to alternative medicine on the Internet. This text is an authoritative guide that will be of extensive and growing use in providing high quality information for individual health professionals, corporations, foundations, international governments, and for all those who are seeking to elicit and sustain optimal health care.

*Kenneth R. Pelletier, PhD, MD(hc)*
*Clinical Professor*
*Complementary Medicine Program*
*University of Maryland School of Medicine*

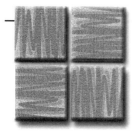

# Preface

At present, there are now over 500 million online Internet users with access to over 3 billion Web pages worldwide. Of these pages, an estimated 2% contain health information, thus resulting in hundreds of millions of pages of health information now accessible on the Web. Recent surveys show that 50% to 75% of World Wide Web users use it to look for health information and those who do so access such information over 3 times a month, making Internet searches for health information one of the most common reasons for going on-line.

In the United States, surveys indicate that between 50 and 100 million adults have searched the World Wide Web for health and medical information. Recent data from the NHS Direct Consumer Health Information Web site *(www.nhsdirect.nhs.uk)* in the UK reveal that the site was accessed 5.2 million times from 171,900 visitors in just 1 month. Responding to this interest in health information is a vast array of health-related Web sites providing information, health care products, services, referrals, and advice. As patients become more involved in their health care decision-making, the balance of knowledge between health care professionals and the public is changing as patients increasingly bring Internet printouts as well as questions about treatment options to the consultation.

This trend is also evident among those seeking information on complementary and alternative medicine (CAM), with the National Center for Complementary and Alternative Medicine's (NCCAM) Web site now receiving over 500,000 hits per month and the Web site *Ask Dr. Weil* receiving 5 million hits per month.

In this book, we hope to enable partnerships between physicians and patients by allowing them to engage in active and productive dialogues regarding these CAM therapies while providing a "roadmap" for finding and evaluating sources of Internet-based information on CAM. There are, however, numerous obstacles to this scenario. These include the sheer volume of health and medical information now available online, the proliferation of dubious and often dangerous information posted on many CAM sites, the limited amount of high quality peer-reviewed research in CAM, inequalities in patient and consumer access to the Internet, and current ethical and legal uncertainties regarding online interactions between physician and patients.

Given that we are still in the midst of this information-driven transformation in health care, it is difficult to foresee what the future holds. It is likely that much of what is required from online information will be similar to that which is required from present conventionally published health and medical information: clear, well-presented

# Complementary Therapies on the Internet

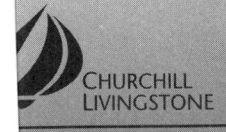

CHURCHILL
LIVINGSTONE

rint of Elsevier Science

# Complementary Therapies
## on the Internet

**William Mac Beckner, BS**
Information Director, Center for Integrative Medicine
University of Maryland School of Medicine
Baltimore, Maryland
USA

**Brian M. Berman, MD**
Director, Center for Integrative Medicine
Professor of Family Medicine
University of Maryland School of Medicine
Baltimore, Maryland
USA

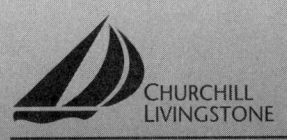

CHURCHILL
LIVINGSTONE

An Imprint of Elsevier Science

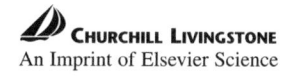
**CHURCHILL LIVINGSTONE**
An Imprint of Elsevier Science

11830 Westline Industrial Drive
St. Louis, Missouri 63146

---

**Notice**

Complementary and alternative medicine is an ever-changing field. Standard safety precautions
must be followed, but as new research and clinical experience broaden our knowledge, change in
treatment and drug therapy may become necessary as appropriate. Readers are advised to check the
most current product information provided by the manufacturer of each drug to be administered
to verify the recommended dose, the method and duration of administration, and contraindications. It is the responsibility of the licensed prescriber, relying on experience and knowledge of the
patient, to determine dosages and the best treatment for each individual patient. Neither the
Publisher nor the authors assume any liability for any injury and/or damage to persons or prop-
erty arising from this publication.

The Publisher

---

**International Standard Book Number 0-443-07067-9**

*Publishing Manager:* Inta Ozols
*Development Editor:* Karen Gilmour
*Publishing Services Manager:* John Rogers
*Project Manager:* Helen Hudlin
*Design:* Dana Peick
*Senior Designer:* Kathi Gosche
*Cover Designer:* Dana Peick

Printed in the United States of America
Last digit is the print number: 9  8  7  6  5  4  3  2  1

and relevant information, with advice on further resources. However, as information technologies continue to evolve, there will be foreseeable advantages to using online health information because of its interactivity, personalization, and the creative ways it offers of managing knowledge.

In deciding to focus on both the tools and resources for locating and evaluating online information regarding CAM therapies, it is our hope that this book will benefit health professionals as well as consumers and patients.

*William Mac Beckner, BS*
*Brian M. Berman, MD*

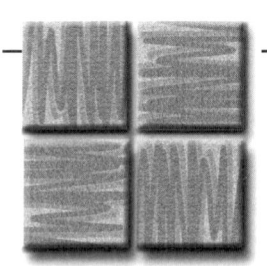

# Acknowledgments

The authors would like to thank the following individuals and institutions for their assistance with this book. Their knowledge, insights, support, and dedication are greatly appreciated.

 ## INDIVIDUALS

Inta Ozols, ELS
Karen Gilmour, ELS
Ken Pelletier, PhD
Judy Emery, PhD
David Riley, MD
Alex Jadad, MD, PhD
Nancy Faass, MSPH

 ## INSTITUTIONS

National Institutes of Health National Center for Complementary and Alternative Medicine
The Cochrane Collection
University of Maryland School of Medicine

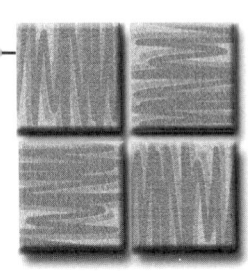

# Contents

1 Complementary and Alternative Medicine and the Internet, *1*

2 Searching the Internet, *15*

3 Searching the Biomedical Literature for Complementary and Alternative Medicine Information, *27*

4 Evaluating Internet Resources in Complementary and Alternative Medicine, *45*

5 Complementary and Alternative Medicine Resources by Modality, *53*

6 Complementary Therapies of the Body, Mind, and Spirit, *71*

7 Complementary and Alternative Medicine Resources for Health Professionals and Researchers, *83*

8 Complementary and Alternative Medicine and Consumer Health Information on the Internet, *117*

9 Legal, Ethical, and Privacy Issues, *131*

10 The Future, *136*

## APPENDICES

1 The Cochrane Collaboration Complementary Medicine Field, *143*

2 Continuing Medical Education in Complementary and Alternative Medicine, *161*

3 Glossary of Complementary and Alternative Medicine Terms, *167*

4 Glossary of Computer and Internet Terms, *173*

# Complementary and Alternative Medicine and the Internet

**Chapter Highlights**
Introduction
History of the Internet
Complementary and Alternative Medicine Defined
Who Uses Complementary and Alternative Medicine
Medical Information on the Internet
Why Patients Use the Internet
Who Uses the Internet for Health Information
Complementary and Alternative Medicine Information
   on the Internet
Conclusion

## INTRODUCTION

Increasingly, individuals around the world are turning to the Internet for health-related knowledge. In the United States, surveys indicate that between 50 million and 70 million adults have searched the World Wide Web for health and medical information.[1] An increasing number of health-related Web sites are now becoming available for up-to-date answers to medical questions. This trend subsequently is affecting the patient-physician relationship.[2,3] With the proliferation of knowledge, the numbers of more informed and educated patients are now greater. Furthermore, of those seeking health information on the Internet, 70% now report that the Internet has influenced their decision about treatment.[4] This trend is evident among those seeking information on complementary therapies and complementary and alternative medicine (CAM), with the National Institutes of Health's National Center for Complementary and Alternative Medicine (NCCAM) Web site now receiving more than 600,000 hits per month and the Web site *Ask Dr. Weil* receiving 2.5 million hits per month (Natural Health Village, accessed December 2001).

Predicting how these trends in health care will evolve is impossible; however, recent developments indicate that these trends will have a profound effect on the way health care consumers, patients, and physicians interact.

With this book the authors hope to guide physicians and patients to equitable access to high-quality information on CAM therapies. In doing so, we hope to enable partnerships between physicians and patients by allowing them to engage in active and productive dialogues regarding these therapies and how to find and evaluate good sources of information on the Internet. Numerous obstacles to this scenario exist, however, and these include the proliferation of dubious and often dangerous information posted on CAM sites, the lack of high-quality peer-reviewed research in CAM, inequalities with access to the Internet, and current ethical and legal uncertainties regarding online interactions between physicians and patients.

Given that we are still in the midst of this information-driven transformation in health care, this book therefore is intended to serve as a guide to CAM health and medical information on the Internet by providing the tools and resources for locating and evaluating online information regarding CAM therapies. Although this book is geared toward the needs of health professionals and providers, the information is certainly relevant to the interests of consumers and patients as well.

##  HISTORY OF THE INTERNET

The Internet began in 1969 when the U.S. Advanced Research Projects Agency (ARPA) began an experiment to link computers across long distances so that they could exchange files and run programs. The network grew slowly at first but then more rapidly. Over the next decade a new computer was added to ARPAnet once every 20 days on average. By the mid-1970s other networks had emerged and began to interlink with ARPAnet. This new network of networks became known as the *internetwork* and soon just *Internet*. The Net, as the network also is called sometimes, continued to expand rapidly as many other host computers from around the world connected to it.

### World Wide Web

The history of the World Wide Web, or Web, begins at **CERN** (Conseil Européen pour la Recherche Nucléaire, or the European Organization for Nuclear Research) **<http://public.web.cern.ch/Public/>** with the work of Tim Berners-Lee and others who brought together the technologies needed to be able to share documents via the Internet by using Web browsers in a multiplatform environment. The technology then evolved from those humble beginnings into the World Wide Web as we know it today **<http://welcome.cern.ch/welcome/gateway.html>** (Fig. 1-1).

### Origins of the Web

Berners-Lee is credited with having created the World Wide Web while he was a researcher at the Laboratory for High-Energy Physics at CERN in Geneva, Switzerland. A tool was needed to enable collaboration between physicists and other researchers in the high-energy physics community.

Berners-Lee wrote a proposal called *HyperText and CERN* and circulated his proposal for comments at CERN in 1989. The proposal **<http://www.w3.org/History/1989/**

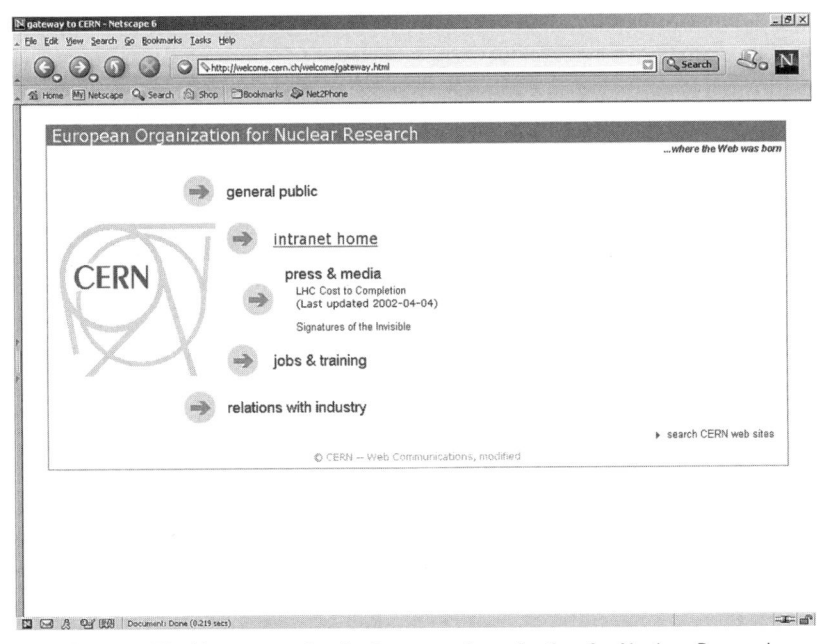

FIG. 1-1 ■ Home page for the European Organization for Nuclear Research.

**proposal>** was the solution to the technologies that would enable collaboration in the high-energy physics community.

In the proposal, three new technologies were introduced. Briefly, they were **HTML** (hypertext markup language) to write the web documents, **HTTP** (hypertext transfer protocol) to transmit the pages, and a **Web browser** client software program to receive and interpret data and display results. An important concept of his proposal was that the **user interface** of the client software program would be consistent across all types of computer platforms so that users could access information from many types of computers worldwide. In May 1991 the first information-sharing system using HTML, HTTP, and a client software program (www) was fully operational and was announced to the public via **UseNET** (the newsgroup), *alt.hypertext,* in August 1991. Early on only one Web server was located at CERN, but by the end of 1992 more than 50 Web servers were located around the world. Many of these earliest Web servers were located at universities or other research centers. By June 1999 more than 720,000 public information servers were in use. As of October of 2001 more than 33 million servers were in use <**http://www.netcraft.co.uk/survey/**> (accessed October 2001).

In 1993, Marc Andreesen was an undergraduate student at the University of Illinois at Urbana-Champaign working on a project for the National Center for Supercomputing Applications (NCSA) when he led a team that developed the graphic interface browser called Mosaic. Persons without computer expertise were able to use the graphic interface and just point and click to navigate the World Wide Web. Since that time the Internet has exploded into a powerful catalyst for global communication. The adoption curve for the Internet has been far more rapid than that of any other established media. The Internet reached 50 million users in 5 years, whereas radio took almost 40 years and television took 13 years to reach similar numbers. According to a Louis Harris poll conducted in 2000, the number of U.S. adults online now totals 60% of the population, with more than 100 million now using the Internet. For those using the Net, sending or receiving e-mail is by a wide margin the most common Internet activity. Thirty-five percent of all those online say they send or receive e-mails "very often," and another 39% do so "often." Worldwide, an average of 250 million users send an average of 8 billion e-mail messages a day.

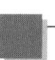 ## COMPLEMENTARY AND ALTERNATIVE MEDICINE DEFINED

Complementary and alternative health care and medical practices are those that are not currently an integral part of conventional medicine. The list of practices considered to be CAM changes continually as CAM practices and therapies that are proved safe and effective become accepted as mainstream health care practices. The practices are defined and organized by the NCCAM into five major domains: (1) alternative medical systems, (2) mind-body interventions, (3) biologically based therapies, (4) manipulative and body-based therapies, and (5) energy therapies (Fig. 1-2 and Box 1-1). The individual systems and treatments composing these categories are too numerous to list in this text, thus only limited number of examples is provided within each.

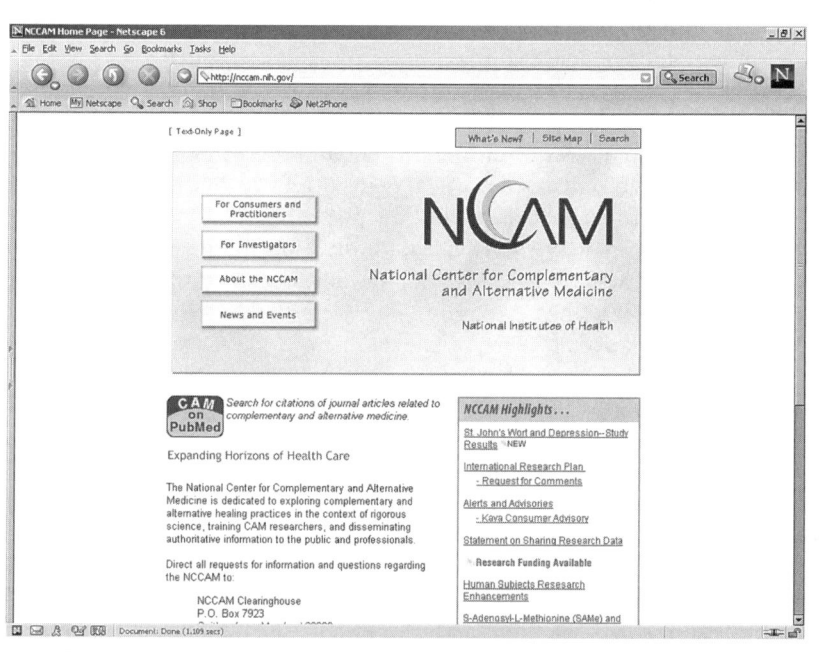

FIG. 1-2   ■   Home page for the National Center for Complementary and Alternative Medicine.

## Alternative Medical Systems

Alternative medical systems involve complete systems of theory and practice that have evolved independent of and often before the conventional biomedical approach. Many are traditional systems of medicine that are practiced by cultures throughout the world and include a number of venerable Asian approaches.

Traditional Asian medicine emphasizes the proper balance or disturbances of *qi* (pronounced *chi*), or vital energy, in health and disease, respectively. Traditional Asian medicine consists of a group of techniques and methods, including acupuncture, herbal medicine, massage, and *qi gong* (a form of energy therapy described more fully in the following text). Acupuncture involves stimulating specific anatomical points in the body for therapeutic purposes, usually by puncturing the skin with a needle.

Ayurveda is traditional system of medicine in India. Ayurvedic medicine (meaning *science of life*) is a comprehensive system of medicine that places equal emphasis on body, mind, and spirit and strives to restore the innate harmony of the individual. Some of the primary Ayurvedic treatments include diet, exercise, meditation, herbs, massage, exposure to sunlight, and controlled breathing. Other traditional medical systems have been developed by Native American, Aboriginal, African, Middle-Eastern, Tibetan, and Central and South American cultures.

Homeopathic and naturopathic medicine are also examples of complete alternative medical systems. Homeopathic medicine is an unconventional Western system based on the principle that "like cures like," that is, that the same substance that in large doses produces the symptoms of an illness, in minute doses cures it. Homeopathic physicians believe that the more dilute the remedy, the greater its potency. Therefore, they use small doses of specially prepared plant extracts and minerals to stimulate the defense mechanisms and healing processes of the body to treat illness.

Naturopathic medicine views disease as a manifestation of alterations in the processes by which the body naturally heals itself and emphasizes health restoration rather than disease treatment. Naturopathic physicians use an array of healing practices, including diet and clinical nutrition; homeopathy; acupuncture; herbal medicine; hydrotherapy (the use of water in a range of temperatures and methods of application); spinal and soft-tissue manipulation; physical therapies involving electric currents, ultrasound, and light therapy; therapeutic counseling; and pharmaceuticals.

---

**Box 1-1  Classification of Complementary and Alternative Medicine***

1. Alternative medical systems
2. Mind-body interventions
3. Biologically based therapies
4. Manipulative and body-based therapies
5. Energy therapies

---

*Classification by the National Center for Complementary and Alternative Medicine, National Institutes of Health.

## Mind–Body Interventions

Mind-body interventions use a variety of techniques designed to facilitate the capacity of the mind to affect bodily function and symptoms. Only a subset of mind-body interventions is considered CAM. On one hand, many interventions that have a well-documented theoretical basis—for example, patient education and cognitive-behavioral approaches—are now considered mainstream. On the other hand, meditation; certain uses of hypnosis; dance, music, and art therapy; and prayer and mental healing are categorized as complementary and alternative.

## Biologically Based Therapies

Biologically based therapies include natural and biologically based practices, interventions, and products, many of which overlap with use of dietary supplements as in conventional medicine. This category includes herbal, special dietary, orthomolecular, and individual biological therapies.

Herbal therapies use individual herbs or mixtures of herbs for therapeutic value. An herb is a plant or plant part that produces and contains chemical substances that act on the body. Special diet therapies, such as those proposed by Drs. Atkins, Ornish, Pritikin, and Weil, are believed to prevent and or control illness and to promote health. Orthomolecular therapies aim to treat disease with varying concentrations of chemicals, such as magnesium, melatonin, and megadoses of vitamins. Biological therapies include, for example, the use of $l$-mandelonitril-$\beta$-glucuronic acid (Laetrile) and shark cartilage to treat cancer and bee pollen to treat autoimmune and inflammatory diseases.

## Manipulative and Body–Based Therapies

Manipulative and body-based therapies include methods based on manipulation or movement of the body. For example, chiropractors focus on the relationship between structure (primarily the spine) and function and how that relationship affects the preservation and restoration of health, using manipulative therapy as an integral treatment tool. Some osteopaths, who place particular emphasis on the musculoskeletal system, believing that all body systems work together and that disturbances in one system may affect function elsewhere in the body, practice osteopathic manipulation. Massage therapists manipulate the soft tissues of the body to normalize those tissues.

## Energy Therapies

Energy therapies focus on energy fields originating within the body (biofields) or those from other sources (electromagnetic fields). Biofield therapies are intended to affect the energy fields, the existence of which is not yet experimentally proven, that surround and penetrate the human body. Some forms of energy therapy manipulate biofields by applying pressure or by manipulating the body by placing the hands in or through these fields. Examples include *qi gong, Reiki,* and Therapeutic Touch. *Qi gong* is a component of traditional Asian medicine that combines movement, meditation, and regulation of breathing to enhance the flow of vital energy (*qi*) in the body to improve blood circulation and to enhance immune function. *Reiki,* the Japanese word representing universal life energy, is based on the belief that by channeling spiritual energy through the practitioner, the spirit is healed and the spirit in turn heals the physical body. Therapeutic Touch is derived from the ancient technique of laying on of hands and is based on the premise that the healing force of the therapist affects the patient's recovery and that healing is promoted when the energies of the body are in balance. By passing their hands over the patient, these healers identify energy imbalances. Bioelectromagnetic-based therapies involve the unconventional use of electromagnetic fields, such as pulsed fields, magnetic fields, or alternating-current or direct-current fields, for example, to treat asthma or cancer or to manage pain and migraine headaches.

In the United Kingdom, the term *complementary medicine* is used broadly, reflecting the perspective that these therapies can be appropriate complements to mainstream care. In the United States, the term *complementary and alternative medicine* is most often used. More than 350 modalities now can be listed under the broad category of CAM. The list of therapies that are considered complementary is likely to evolve continually as CAM modalities that are proved safe and effective become accepted as mainstream health care practice.

## Trends in Integrative Medicine

Beginning in 1996 the term *integrative medicine* came into wider use in the medical literature. In a growing trend, some alternative therapies are being integrated into clinical medicine in the United States. In 1998 the *Journal of the American Medical Association* proposed the development of "one medicine"—a guarded invitation to include select alternative therapies in biomedicine—predicated on an evidence-based approach.[5] Since that time multiple research efforts have sought to assess these therapies from the perspectives of efficacy, cost, third-party reimbursement, credentialing, licensing, and other criteria. These initiatives primarily have involved the National Institutes of Health in partnership with many academic institutions. In addition, numerous conferences now are sponsored annually by prestigious universities such as Harvard, Stanford, and Columbia. More recently, in Janaury, 2002, twelve leading medical institutions formed the Association of Academic Health Centers for Integrative Medicine. The mission of the association is to help transform health care through rigorous scientific studies, new models of clinical care, and innovative educational programs that integrate biomedicine while respecting the complexity of human beings, the intrinsic nature of healing, and the rich diversity of therapeutic systems.

The growing interest in integrative medicine by business organizations is reflected in an annual summit on the development of a business model for integrative medicine sponsored by industry leaders that brings together major stakeholders, including researchers, policy makers, and health insurers.

 WHO USES COMPLEMENTARY AND ALTERNATIVE MEDICINE

The best data on rates of use of complementary and alternative therapies comes from two surveys conducted by Eisenberg and others in 1990 and 1997.[6,7] Data extrapo-

 **TABLE 1-1** National Projections of Expenditures for Complementary and Alternative Medicine[7]

| SOURCE OF PAYMENT AND TYPE OF EXPENSE | ESTIMATED RANGE OF EXPENDITURES ON CAM (IN BILLIONS OF DOLLARS) | |
| --- | --- | --- |
| | 1990 | 1997 |
| Reimbursed expenditures: CAM professional services; 15 therapies | $7.4 to $11.6 | $9 to $13.1 |
| Out-of-pocket expenditures: CAM professional services; 15 therapies | $7.2 to $11 | $12.2 to $19.6 |
| Out-of-pocket expenditures spent on self-care: megavitamins, diet products, herbal medicine, books, classes, equipment | – | $14.8 |
| Total CAM expenditures | $14.6 to $22.6 | $36 to $47.5 |

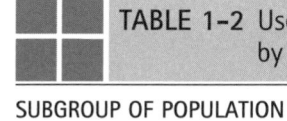 **TABLE 1-2** Use of Complementary and Alternative Medicine by Population Subgroup[8]

| SUBGROUP OF POPULATION | CAM USE |
| --- | --- |
| "Cultural creatives" (23% of the U.S. population) | 55% |
| Respondents with graduate degrees | 50% |
| Respondents who maintain a holistic philosophy | 46% |
| Respondents earning $40,000 or more | 44% |

**TABLE 1-3** Use of Complementary and Alternative Medicine by Population Subset[8]

| SUBSET OF POPULATION | CAM USE |
| --- | --- |
| Respondents with some college | 50.6% |
| Respondents 25 to 49 years old | 50.1% |
| Female respondents | 48.9% |
| Respondents with incomes above $50,000 | 48.1% |

lated from the 1990 telephone survey of approximately 1600 respondents, representative of all social and economic groups, found that about one third of all Americans had used complementary and alternative therapies in that year. Almost all of those surveyed were also currently under conventional care. However, about 90% referred themselves to CAM providers, and only one out of four told their physicians they did so.[6] A repeat of this survey in 1997 with more than 2000 respondents showed a dramatic increase in CAM use to 42%. Out-of-pocket expenditures were equal to out-of-pocket medical expenditures. CAM expenditures for 1997 were esti-

TABLE 1-4  Conditions Treated by Complementary and Alternative Medicine Therapies and Percentage of Use Reported by Respondents

| CONDITION | DATA FROM EISENBERG AND OTHERS, 1997[7] | DATA FROM ASTIN, 1997[8] |
|---|---|---|
| Neck conditions | 57% | — |
| Back conditions | 47.6% | — |
| Anxiety | 42.7% | 31% |
| Depression | 40.9% | 31% |
| Chronic pain | — | 37% |
| Headaches | 32.2% | 24% |
| Digestive disorders | 27.3% | — |
| Fatigue | 27% | — |
| Arthritis/rheumatism | 26.7% | 25% |
| Insomnia | 26.4% | — |
| Addictions | — | 25% |
| Sprains and strains | 23.6% | 26% |

mated at $36 billion to $47.5 billion. Among certain subsets of the population, Eisenberg found that CAM use approached 50%[7] (Table 1-1).

In the study by Astin,[8] a written survey was mailed to individuals randomly selected from a nationally representative panel. The overall projection was CAM use by about 40% of the population. Astin's survey defined and identified respondents by demographics and by subculture (Table 1-2). In Astin's research, groups reporting highest use included those with some college education and those identified as "cultural creatives" (Tables 1-2 and 1-3).

Internationally, similar and higher rates of CAM use can be found in surveys performed in Europe, Australia, Japan, Australia, and other countries. In the United Kingdom, Germany, and France, a parity of use exists between mainstream and complementary therapies, according to several studies.[9-11] In the United Kingdom, research indicates that 40% of general practitioners offer their patients access to complementary medicine, and the National Health Service currently is providing many of these therapies through the health care system. Chiropractic and osteopathy are the two treatments most frequently used, particularly for lower back pain.[12] Massage, acupuncture, and even spiritual healing also are providing patients with greater choices.

## Why Patients Use Complementary and Alternative Medicine

The predominant reason for patient use of complementary therapies is to alleviate chronic illness and stress-related conditions such as back problems, arthritis, depression, hypertension, digestive disorders, cancer, and autoimmune syndrome (Table 1-4). Patients are attracted to complementary therapies because these modalities are part of their social network or because they are drawn to the philosophy and beliefs of whole-person care.[8] Other studies suggest that patients use CAM because they want to function as active participants in their own health care[7] or because they are not satisfied with the process and results of conventional care.[13] Surveys have found that about 50% of cancer and human immunodeficiency virus (HIV) patients will use complementary therapies at some point in their illness.[14] In short, two of the primary patient motivations for using CAM are efforts in prevention and wellness and in the treatment of chronic illness.

### Therapeutic Modalities Used

Some of the most frequently used complementary therapies include special diet, exercise, and relaxation techniques. The most frequently used modalities involving treatment by a practitioner are chiropractic, massage, self-help groups, and imagery. Other frequently used modalities include megavitamin therapy and herbal medicine (Table 1-5).

 MEDICAL INFORMATION ON THE INTERNET

The Internet, via the World Wide Web, provides for an unprecedented exchange of medical information. More and more health care providers are interacting with their colleagues via e-mail and are interested in using e-mail and the Web to interact with patients, to locate the most current literature on the effectiveness of specific treatments, and to conduct research themselves, sometimes in collaboration with colleagues worldwide.

 WHY PATIENTS USE THE INTERNET

Data from the Pew Internet and American Life report gives abundant evidence that the Internet has become a valued source of health care information for a substantial

| TABLE 1-5 Prevalence and Frequency of Use of Alternative Therapies in the United States, 1997[7] | | | |
|---|---|---|---|
| THERAPY | TOTAL ESTIMATED ANNUAL VISITS (IN MILLIONS) | NUMBER OF VISITS PER THOUSAND MEMBERS OF THE U.S. POPULATION | MEAN NUMBER OF VISITS PER USER ANNUALLY |
| Chiropractic | 192 | 969.1 | 9.8 |
| Massage | 114 | 574.4 | 8.4 |
| Self-help groups | 80 | 402.8 | 18.9 |
| Commercial diet | 27 | 138.8 | 7.3 |
| Imagery | 22 | 114.3 | 11 |
| Megavitamins | 22 | 112.1 | Not available |
| Herbal medicine | 10 | 53 | 2.9 |
| Acupuncture | 5 | 27.2 | 3.1 |
| Hypnotherapy | 4 | 21.1 | 1.6 |
| Biofeedback | 4 | 19.5 | 3.6 |

number of Internet users. Fifty-two million adult Americans, 55% of the Internet-user population, have turned to Internet sources to seek health information.[1] Patients and their families are using the Internet to help with many aspects of care, but they are most likely to have sought material about the options they have for battling illnesses and the prognoses for those illnesses.

In addition, they investigate how to participate in clinical trials for new drugs; they examine reports on the course of diseases; they buy vitamins, download recipes for fat-free foods, use calorie calculators, and search for ways to develop "washboard abs." Furthermore, they check report cards for hospitals, doctors, and health insurers. Some support each other through disease-specific bulletin boards and trade ideas about how to deal with symptoms within support groups. These activities are taking place in an environment where the burden of responsibility in the health care system has shifted more to patients as health maintenance organizations and tighter insurance rules have compelled them to take more assertive roles in their own care. A typical doctor's visit reportedly has shrunk to less than 15 minutes, and many patients leave a physician's office without getting answers to all the questions they have. One 1999 survey by Yankelovich Monitor[15] <**http://www.yankelovich.com**> found that half or more of Americans are not satisfied with the availability of their doctors and are not satisfied with the duration of their meetings with their doctors. Not surprisingly, many Internet users have turned to the Web to provide the information they find hard to get from their caregivers and because they increasingly are interested in participating in what the medical community calls shared decision making.

To put things in perspective, Table 1-6 shows how searches for health information compare with use rates for other popular online activities.

## WHO USES THE INTERNET FOR HEALTH INFORMATION

According to the Pew report, less-healthy persons are more likely to seek such information frequently: 32% of those who say they are in less than excellent health go online once per week, compared with 23% of those who say they are in excellent health. On a typical day online, more than 5.5 million Americans search the Internet for health information.[1]

More women than men seek health information. Sixty-three percent of women with Internet access have sought health information, whereas 46% of men with

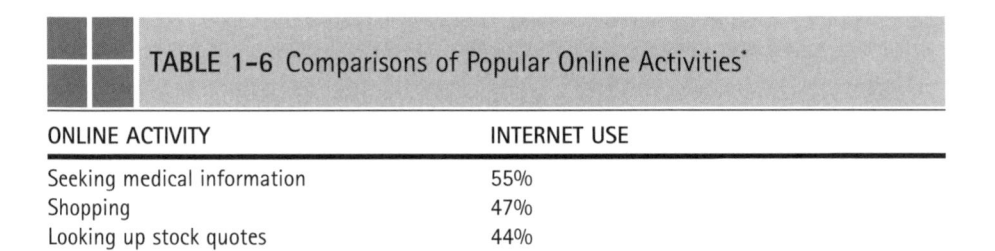

**TABLE 1-6** Comparisons of Popular Online Activities*

| ONLINE ACTIVITY | INTERNET USE |
| --- | --- |
| Seeking medical information | 55% |
| Shopping | 47% |
| Looking up stock quotes | 44% |
| Checking sports scores | 36% |

*From Pew Internet and American Life Project survey, July–August 2000.

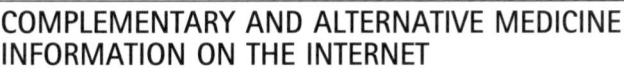

| TABLE 1-7 Percentage of Internet Users Who Seek Medical Information Online, by Subgroup* | |
| --- | --- |
| SUBGROUP | USE |
| All Internet users | 55% |
| Online women | 63% |
| Online men | 46% |
| Veteran users (3 or more years) | 59% |
| New users (less than 6 months) | 47% |
| Online parents | 59% |
| Online non-parents | 52% |

*From Pew Internet and American Life Project survey, July-August 2000.

Internet access have done so. Health information seekers are proportionally more middle-aged than very young or old, with the highest proportions of usage showing up in those between the ages of 30 and 64. Two thirds of women between the ages of 30 and 49 who have Internet access have gone online to get health or medical information. The other demographic trait that distinguishes health information seekers is their level of experience with the Internet. The longer someone has had access to the Internet, the more likely that person has gotten medical information. Some 59% of those with 3 years of Internet experience have sought medical information, compared with 47% of those who first went online within the past 6 months[1] (Table 1-7).

In the survey, 91% of health information seekers reported they were covered by health insurance and the rest said they were not covered, which means health information seekers are more likely to have insurance than are members of the general U.S. population. The rest of the demographic story about health information seekers is notable for what *does not occur*. In contrast to many other online activities, seeking health information is equally compelling to all racial and ethnic groups. Similarly, income has no major effect on this activity. The likelihood that someone has gotten health information does not correlate with household income. Compared with online auctions or online banking, for example, the search for health information is a popular activity with newcomers to the Internet, and they are more likely to be members of minority groups and those from households with incomes under $50,000.

## COMPLEMENTARY AND ALTERNATIVE MEDICINE INFORMATION ON THE INTERNET

The data examined indicate apparently that, for now, patients are using the Internet to learn more about their health conditions, not only those who use alternative therapies but also those who are pursuing conventional therapies.[16] Interest in Internet-based CAM information is evidenced by the tremendous Internet traffic to the

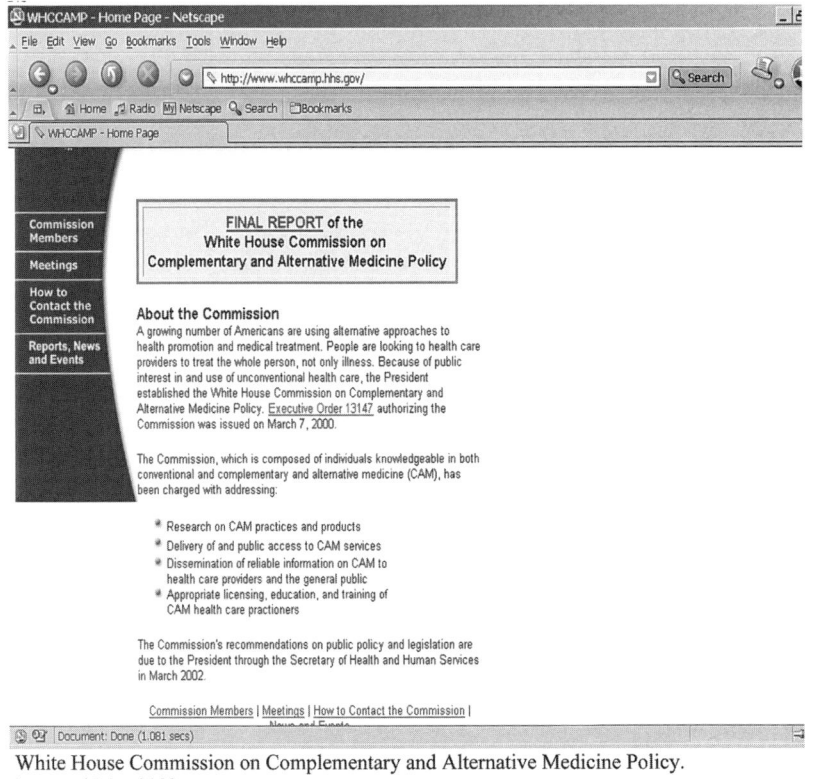

White House Commission on Complementary and Alternative Medicine Policy.
Accessed May 2002.

**FIG. 1-3** ■  Final report of the White House Commission on Complementary and Alternative Medicine Policy.

National Institutes of Health National Center for Complementary and Alternative Medicine Web site **<http://www.nccam.nih.gov>**, which receives more than 600,000 hits per month (Straus NCRR Testimony; White House Commission Meeting Transcript, March 26, 2001 **<http://www.whccamp.hhs.gov/meetings/ transcript_3_26_01v1p1.html>**) (Fig. 1-3).

## 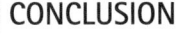 CONCLUSION

In this chapter we have discussed the origin of the Internet and how it has developed into the World Wide Web of today. We defined and described how patients increasingly are using the Web for health and medical information and the growing interest in CAM by patients who are using the Internet to access health information. In Chapter 2 we will discuss how the Internet is structured and how to navigate and search the Web for specific medical and CAM information.

## References

1. Fox SR: *The Pew Internet and American Life Project: the online health care revolution: how the Web helps Americans take better care of themselves*, November 26, 2000, The Pew Charitable Trust.
2. Podolsky DK: Patients, gastroenterologists, and the World Wide Web, *Gastroenterology* 114(1):5, 1998.
3. McLellan MF: Are you using the Internet for nursing? *AWHONN Lifelines* 1(3):20, June, 1997 (miscellaneous).
4. Berland GK and others: Health information on the Internet: accessibility, quality, and readability in English and Spanish, *JAMA* 285(20):2612-2621, 2001.
5. Fontanarosa PB, Lundberg GD: Alternative medicine meets science, *JAMA* 280(18):1618-1619, 1998.
6. Eisenberg DM and others: Unconventional medicine in the United States. Prevalence, costs, and patterns of use, *N Engl J Med* 328(4):246-252, 1993.
7. Eisenberg DM and others: Trends in alternative medicine use in the United States, 1990-1997: results of a follow-up national survey, *JAMA* 280(18):1569-1575, 1998.
8. Astin JA: Why patients use alternative medicine: results of a national study, *JAMA* 279(19):1548-1553, 1998.
9. MacLennan AH, Wilson DH, Taylor AW: Prevalence and cost of alternative medicine in Australia, *Lancet* 347(9001):569-573, 1996.
10. Fisher P, Ward A: Complementary medicine in Europe, *BMJ* 309(6947):107-111, 1994.
11. Fulder SJ, Munro RE: Complementary medicine in the United Kingdom: patients, practitioners, and consultations, *Lancet* 2(8454):542-545, 1985.
12. Vickers A: Reflections on complementary medicine research in the UK, *Complement Ther Med* 7(4):199-200, 1999.
13. Furnham A, Forey J: The attitudes, behaviors, and beliefs of patients of conventional vs. complementary (alternative) medicine, *J Clin Psychol* 50(3):458-469, 1994.
14. McGinnis LS: Alternative therapies, 1990: an overview, *Cancer* 67(suppl 6):1788-1792, 1991.
15. Yankelovich Monitor: *State of the Consumer Report. Consumers take health into their own hands, http://www.yankelovich.com/, 2001.*
16. Penson RT and others: Complementary, alternative, integrative, or unconventional medicine? *Oncologist* 6(5):463-473, 2001.

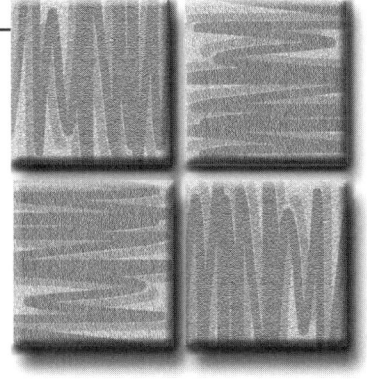

# Searching the Internet

**Chapter Highlights**
Introduction
Getting the Information You Want
Defining the Question
Choosing Search Tools and Methods
Conducting and Refining Searches
Interpreting the Results
Conclusion

## INTRODUCTION

Finding the Web documents and Web pages that you want can be easy or seem impossibly difficult in part because of the sheer size of the World Wide Web, which currently is estimated to contain 3 billion documents, and because the Web is not indexed in any standard vocabulary. Unlike library catalogs that use standardized Library of Congress subject headings, on the Web you need to make an educated guess as to what words will be in the pages you want to find or what subject terms were chosen by the creator of the Web page or site covering some topic.

Additionally, searching the Web directly is not possible. The Web is the totality of all the Web pages that reside on computers (called *servers*) all over the world. A search via the Internet cannot find or go to them all directly. What you are able to do through your computer is access one or more of many intermediate search tools now available. You search the database or collection of sites of the search tool—a small subset of the entire World Wide Web. The search tool provides you with hypertext links with uniform resource locators (URLs) to other pages. You click on these links and retrieve documents, images, sound, and more from individual servers around the world. No means exists for anyone to search the entire Web, and any search tool that claims to offer such is distorting the truth.

In health care an exponential growth of formal research studies is now generating new scientific information at the rate of 2 million biomedical articles per year published in 20,000 journals. Finding valid health and medical information on the

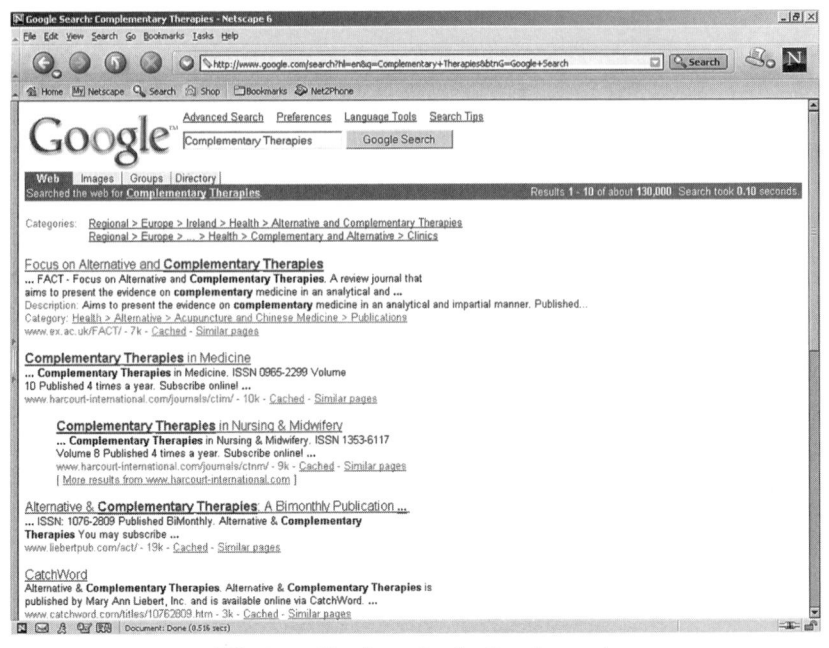

**FIG. 2-1** ■ Example of a Google search.

Internet can be difficult because of the tremendous size of the Internet (Fig. 2-1) and lack of quality standards for the hundreds of millions of pages of health information now available. As a result, what many health professionals are discovering is a disturbing and even frightening overload of information that is easy to access but increasingly difficult to evaluate. For example, if you enter the search term "*alternative medicine*" in the Google search engine, you will retrieve more than 600,000 hits. Furthermore, if you search for "*alternative medicine*" *AND* "*miracle cancer cure,*" you retrieve more than 1400 hits (Google search, October 2001). This tremendous volume of information ranges from high-quality synopses of systematic reviews to sites that promote questionable, useless, or dangerous therapies, treatments, and products.

Clearly, many ways exist to find information on the Internet. However, because of the more than 2 billion indexed pages (Google), searching can be an arduous and time-consuming task to filter through all the information available on the Internet. Using tools such as Internet guides, directories, and search engines can assist health professionals, patients, and consumers in their search for health information. However, searching for and locating health information are only starting points, after which the users themselves must choose the appropriate resources and information to guide their decisions.

## ■ GETTING THE INFORMATION YOU WANT

In designing a good Internet search, a deliberate, structured approach to finding information on the Web typically includes four elements:

1.  Defining the question

2. Choosing search tools and methods
3. Conducting and refining searches
4. Interpreting the results

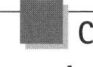 DEFINING THE QUESTION

Are you looking for a specific fact or for a particular Web site? Or is your intent to browse around, grazing the Web for samples of information that might or might not fill the gaps in the puzzle you are assembling? Do you want recommendations or reviews by experts? Or perhaps you are a student, a scientist, or an attorney and need everything available on a particular subject? As you can see, the type of search and the nature and quantity of results are different in each of these types of searches. You should have a clear idea before you begin your search whether you are trying to locate, browse, consult, or capture all the available data. This will help you select an appropriate search tool and save time.

CHOOSING SEARCH TOOLS AND METHODS

A **search tool** is a computer program that performs searches. A **search method** is the way a search tool requests and retrieves information from its Web site. A search begins at the Web site of the search tool, reached by means of its address or URL. Each search tool Web site comprises a store of information called a database. This database has links to other databases at other Web sites, and the other Web sites have links to still other Web sites, and so on. Thus each search tool has extended search capabilities by means of a worldwide system of links.

Essentially four types of search tools are available, each of which has its own search method. The following discussion describes these search tools and then suggests exercises for achieving a familiarity with their use.

1. A **directory search tool** searches for information by subject matter. The search is hierarchical and starts with a general subject heading and follows with a succession of increasingly more specific sub-headings. The search method used is known as a **subject search.**

   ■ *Tip:* You choose a subject search when you want general information on a subject or topic. Often you can find links in the references provided that will lead to specific information you want.

   ■ *Advantage:* The directory search tool is easy to use. Also, information placed in its database is reviewed and indexed first by skilled persons to ensure its value.

   ■ *Disadvantage:* Because directory reviews and indexing are so time consuming, the number of reviews is limited. Thus directory databases are comparatively small and their updating frequency is low. Also, descriptive information about each site is limited and general.

2. A **search engine tool** searches for information through use of keywords and responds with a list of references or hits. The search method used is known as a **keyword search.**

- *Tip:* You choose a keyword search to obtain specific information because the extensive database is likely to contain the information sought.
- *Advantage:* The information content or database of a search engine tool is substantially larger and more current than that of a directory search tool.
- *Disadvantage:* The search engine tool is not exacting in the way it indexes and retrieves information in its database, which makes finding relevant documents more difficult.

Keyword searches require far more explanation than subject searches because of their broader scope and greater complexity.

3. A **directory with search engine** uses the subject and keyword search methods interactively as described previously. In the directory search, the search follows the directory path through increasingly more specific subject matter. At each stop along the path, a search engine option is provided to enable the searcher to convert to a keyword search. The subject and keyword searches are thus said to be **coordinated.** The further down the path the keyword search is made, the narrower the search field is and the fewer and more relevant the hits are.
   - *Tip:* You use a coordinated search when you are uncertain whether a subject or keyword search will provide the best results.
   - *Advantage:* The coordinated search has the capability to narrow the search field to obtain better results.
   - *Disadvantage:* This search method may not succeed for difficult searches.

Some search tools use search engine and directory searches independently. They are said to be **noncoordinated.**

4. A **multiengine search tool** (sometimes called a **metasearch**) uses a number of search engines in parallel. The search is conducted via keywords using commonly used operators or plain language. The search then lists the hits by search engine used or by integrating the results into a single listing.
   - *Tip:* You use the metasearch to speed up the search process and to avoid redundant hits.
   - *Advantage:* The metasearch tolerates imprecise search questions and provides fewer hits of likely greater relevance.
   - *Disadvantage:* The metasearch is not as effective as a search engine for difficult searches.

A search tool uses a computer program to access Web sites and retrieve information. Each search tool is owned by a single entity, such as person, company, or organization, which operates the search tool from a master computer. When you use a search tool, your request travels to the search tool Web site, which conducts a search of its database and directs the response to your computer.

Box 2-1 lists preferred search tools, which are some of the best search tools presently available on the Web. As a group, these search engines and directories were chosen because they provide diversity and depth.

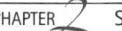 *Box* 2-1  Preferred Search Tools

**DIRECTORY (SUBJECT SEARCH)**

| | |
|---|---|
| Encyclopedia Britannica | Yahoo |
| Looksmart | About.com |

**SEARCH ENGINE (KEYWORD SEARCH)**

| | | |
|---|---|---|
| AltaVista | HotBot | Fast |
| Google | Infoseek | OneKey |
| Excite | Northern Light | Snap |

**MULTIENGINE (METASEARCH)**

| | |
|---|---|
| Dogpile | Metacrawler |
| Mamma | Savvy Search |

##  CONDUCTING AND REFINING SEARCHES

### Simple Searches

For beginners and nonexperts, the operators used in simple searches are sufficient for composing most all queries. You use them in whatever combination provides the best definition. The examples shown are illustrative and are not necessarily ideal queries.

#### Plus and Minus

Use a plus sign (+) before a query term to require its presence in the Web document sought.

Example: **+ herbal + medicine + safety**

This query gives an enormous number of hits because each term can be anywhere in the document and is not related necessarily to any other. Nonetheless, because the hits are ranked, the highest-ranking ones should contain all the terms and therefore likely should produce relevant documents.

Use the minus sign (hyphen) similarly to prohibit the use of a term. This technique is particular useful when you wish to exclude irrelevant subject matter. The following query example searches for alternative medicine while limiting or excluding sites with products claiming miracle cures.

Example: **+ "alternative medicine" − "miracle cure" − "product"**

#### Stemming

To include variations of a keyword, you use the wild card symbol (* or asterisk) after the stem of the word. This broadens a search to retrieve documents that otherwise would be missed.

Example: **Acu***

This search includes the words *acupuncture, acupressure,* and a*cupoint.* You should not use stemming if too many irrelevant terms are introduced.

### Phrases

A phrase is a sequence of words that has a particular meaning and is formed by enclosure within double quotation marks. A phrase is treated as a single term and usually is searched as such.
Example: **"alternative medicine"**
If a query asks for *alternative medicine* rather than *"alternative medicine,"* the responses will be for the words *alternative* and *medicine* separately, in addition to the coupled words. This increases the number of irrelevant hits.
You should use phrases appropriately whenever you can; they are one of the most effective means of sharpening meaning and narrowing a search.
Example: + **"research methods"** + **"complementary medicine"**
The previous example is a much more definitive query than the following one:
Example: + **research** + **methods** + **complementary** + **medicine**

### Case Sensitive

Capitalization rules apply to proper names as taught in English classes. However, treating a multiple-word name as a phrase by enclosing it within double quotation marks is more definitive.
Example: **"holistic health care directory"**

## Advanced Searches

Each search tool tends to devise and organize its operators differently. An advanced search includes simple and advanced operators, much like that of AltaVista.

### Boolean

Although Boolean operators are somewhat complex, most professionals prefer them because they can compose more precise queries.
AND does not promise any association between terms and thus broadens a search. When unrestricted, AND can produce an enormous number of hits.
Complications can occur when query terms have no operators between them. Some search engines assume AND as the default between the terms, whereas others assume NEAR. Therefore, using a plus sign (+) before each term rather than leaving a space is more exact.
NEAR generally indicates that the query terms it connects are within about two to 25 words of each other, depending on the search engine. This proximity makes finding an association between the terms more likely, thereby helping to narrow the search.
OR broadens a search and is best used in a phrase to designate synonyms.
Example: **"complementary medicine OR alternative medicine OR integrative medicine"**
Synonyms significantly improve the odds of finding documents you want. The more synonyms you use, the more weight is given to their importance.

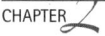

NOT excludes even a single use of the term in the document and is used most suitably to reduce a large number of irrelevant hits when other measures have failed. Example: **"herbs NOT garden"**

### Parentheses

You should enclose phrases within parentheses (called *nesting*) to narrow a search further, especially when unlike operators are used in the query.
Example: **search + (research AND alternative medicine) + ("grants AND funding")**
    In the search process, phrases are searched before the other terms in the query, which narrows the search area for the non-phrase terms.

### Fields

Many fields are available, but the two you are most likely to find useful are title and URL fields. When you think a term is likely to be in a particular field, you should use the term in that query. The field symbol that precedes the query may differ among search engines. For example, the symbol can be *title* or *t* or *url* or *u*.
Example: **title:"search CAM"**
    Field choices usually are found in the vicinity of the query box or are reached by clicking an appropriate link.

## Refining Results

Most search engines that use advanced searches offer options for refining your query to improve the results. This can be helpful in improving your search. The options vary among the search engines and are straightforward to use. You should start using advanced operators when you can do so comfortably. Some, you will find, are easy to apply and can be helpful in improving results when you are searching for obscure information.

## Query Composition Guides

Despite the differences in the way search engines select, index, and retrieve documents, some common guides exist to help compose a query.

- You should be as specific and complete as you can in selecting your keywords; they are critical to the success of your search.
- When possible, you should use uncommon or unique terms, for they are less likely to be ignored or filtered. You should avoid adjectives and adverbs unless they are part of a phrase; by themselves they do not convey much meaning.
- You should arrange your terms in a series from the most general to the most specific; it makes for a more effective search.
- When using the same query for multiple searches, you should use suitable, advanced operators. Most search engines support advanced operators to advantage, although some may ignore them or apply them differently.
- When you have located a good site about your topic, you should see whether the site has links to other sites. Sometimes an important document is found this way. The site also may contain keywords that can improve a query.

- You should use the refined drop-down lists when offered. They are a simple way to narrow your search.
- You should avoid misspellings, redundant terms, and complicated query structures.

### Search Problems and Remedies

Even when your query is well defined, a search engine at times returns totally irrelevant responses. The following explains some of the causes and suggests remedies you can try.

1. Your query terms do not have a counterpart in the index of the search engine.

   **Cause:** You may have insufficient understanding of the composing criteria of the search engine.

   *Remedy: You should study the help section of the search engine and recompose your query accordingly.*

2. The search engine has failed to index significant keywords while spidering the Internet.

   **Cause:** The search engine uses abbreviated rather than full-word spidering in creating and maintaining its database. Therefore, the engine can miss important keywords because of their infrequent use or unfavorable location in the document.

   *Remedy: You should use a search engine that uses full-word spidering, such as AltaVista, HotBot, Excite, or Infoseek.*

3. The search engine filters out or ignores important keywords used in your query. This corrupts the meaning of the query, resulting in irrelevant results.

   **Cause:** Search engines with large databases ignore or filter a few commonly used words because of the enormous amount of processing they require. The problem arises when a query keyword you use is also the designated common word of the search engine (for example, *Internet, computer,* and *Web*).

   *Remedies: You should use a search engine with a moderate-sized database such as Infoseek, Excite, or Snap. Another approach is to use a subject search tool having a large database. Yahoo is recommended because of its large subject index and the keyword search option it provides.*

At times, despite all the skills you can apply, you still may not be able to find the document you want. Although the information indexed in the Web is enormous, it is not necessarily complete, up to date, or reasonably accessible. Search tools are addressing the problem, including that created by the recent unprecedented growth of Web pages. But despite its less than perfect performance, the Internet remains a remarkable source of information.

### Specific Search Engines

How do various search engines index the Web, how do they search the Web, and how do they prioritize Web sites? The process involves sophisticated algorithms, with some search engines being geared toward dot-coms—toward products and services—

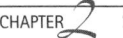

whereas others use algorithms that allow them to measure the number of inbound links or outbound links in the Web sites that are being searched. This is comparable to measuring impact factor on journals: the more well-referenced a Web site is, the higher it ranks in a Google search, for example. Search strategy involves evaluating the type of search engine, how it interfaces with the Web, whether it indexes the entire Web, and more importantly, how the search engine brings the information to you and what protocol it uses.

In designing your search, you should consider the general design and function of the major search sites. Becoming familiar with their advanced options is also helpful to focus searches. Similarly, knowing the features or options each search site uses is helpful to differentiate it from the others. The following is a current sample of Internet search engines and directories with their differentiating characteristics.

### Achoo

*Home page address:* <http://www.achoo.com/main.asp>
*Help page address:* <http://www.achoo.com/help/default.asp>
*Advanced query:* <http://www.achoo.com/search/default.asp>
*Search method:* Primarily keyword, with a subject option that draws on subject directories. Achoo also provides popular sites on its home page under "Specialty Searches."
*Database:* Health care database on the Internet for Web sites on specific topics. The database is organized by keyword, geographical location, and information type.
*Operators:* Achoo uses advanced search with simple and advanced operators.
*Features:* Health care focus gateway including four focus areas: search engine, news, commerce, and disease-oriented online communities.

### AltaVista

*Home page address:* <http://www.altavista.com/>
*Help page address, simple query:* <http://www.altavista.com/sites/help>
*Advanced query:* <http://www.altavista.com/sites/search/adv>
*Search method:* Primarily keyword, with a subject option that draws on LookSmart subject directories. AltaVista also provides popular sites on its home page under "Specialty Searches."
*Database:* Full text with one of the largest and most inclusive directory indexes.
*Operators:* AltaVista uses advanced search with simple and advanced operators. The latter operators are comprehensive and sophisticated.
*Features:* AltaVista provides ways of narrowing a search; can limit a search by date and retrieve references by last date modified; and translates text into a number of languages. AltaVista also uses Ask Jeeves, which accepts queries in simple question form and can be configured to filter objectionable material from searches.
*Comments:* AltaVista is a leading search engine and has one of the largest databases and most effective search systems. If not used properly, AltaVista can produce an extraordinary number of irrelevant hits. AltaVista serves as the default search engine for LookSmart and Britannica Internet Guide.

## Excite

*Home page address:* <http://www.excite.com/>
*Help page address:* <http://www.excite.com/Info/searching.html?a-n-t>
*Search method:* Primarily keyword with subject option. Excite provides long lists of popular sites under several headings.
*Database:* Full-text search of about 75 million documents.
*Operators:* Excite supports simple and advanced searches.
*Features:* Excite offers keyword searches for literal or concept queries but does better with concept searches. Concept search is the default. (A concept search looks for ideas related to a literal query.) Use of Boolean operators turns off concept searching. The channel sites in Excite are approved by editors and sometimes have reviews.
*Comments:* Excite is easy to use, its headings and links are well organized, and the instructions for its use are presented clearly. Excite includes current news-related items with the search results. Excite runs Webcrawler as an independent metasearch tool.

## Google

*Home page address:* <http://www.google.com/>
*Help page address:* <http://www.google.com/help.html>
*Advanced query:* <http://www.google.com/advanced_search?>
*Search method:* Primarily keyword. Google also provides a Web directory by major topic heading. By selecting "I'm feeling lucky" as an option, you may limit the search to the most relevant site.
*Database:* More than 2 billion pages.
*Operators:* "Simple Search" operators are suitable. The plus operator (+) is automatic.
*Features:* Google returns only pages that match all the terms in the query. Google also tries to return results where the terms are in proximity, has an image search engine and content filters, and ranks hits based on their use popularity.
*Comments:* Google has a sophisticated database yet provides an uncluttered and easy-to-use format. Google can limit searches to particular categories, such as government- and Linux-related sites.

## Northern Light

*Home page address:* <http://www.northernlight.com/>
*Help page address:* <http://www.northernlight.com/docs/search_help_optimize.html>
*Search method:* Primarily subject with auxiliary keyword.
*Database:* Among the largest.
*Operators:* Northern Light supports "Simple Search" operators.
*Features:* Northern Light provides a special collection listing by subject derived from 1800 journals, reviews, books, magazines, and news wires. These documents are not readily accessible to other search engine robots. Searching is free, and the cost to use the database is modest.
*Comments:* Northern Light is a well-organized search tool and searches the Web and the special collection separately.

### Yahoo

*Home page address:* <http://www.yahoo.com/>

*Help page address:* <http://www.yahoo.com/docs/info/help.html>

*Frequently asked questions:* <http://www.yahoo.com/docs/info/faq.html>

*Search method:* Primarily subject with coordinated keyword option. In keyword searches, Yahoo selects only sites that contain all search words. If no exact match is found, Yahoo switches automatically to Inktomi.

*Database:* Yahoo reviews its own keyword database and has at least 1 million subject sites listed.

*Operators:* When a search defaults to the Inktomi search tool, "Simple Search" and "Advanced Search" are applicable.

*Features:* Yahoo can search by title (t) and URL (u) and lists popular sites.

*Comments:* Yahoo has the largest subject database on the Web. Its headings and links are well organized and easy to use. Yahoo is a great place for beginners to originate a search.

## INTERPRETING THE RESULTS

Defining your search and selecting the appropriate search tool will take you a long way toward getting good search results. The final step in the process is to take a critical look at your results *before* you examine pages in detail. You should look at three key areas as you make your assessment.

- *Title.* Titles in search results are the actual links to documents. Does the title contain at least one of your search keywords? Are the other keywords in the title relevant to your search, or are they an amalgam of words designed to catch the attention of indexing spiders? A descriptive title usually, but not always, can be one of the best indicators that you have found what you are seeking. If a page has no title, Infoseek and Lycos use the first line of text on the page, and the other search engines display the URL or indicate that no title was available.
- *Page description.* Intuitively, the description should be the most useful part of a search result. But each search engine creates descriptions differently. AltaVista, HotBot, Infoseek, and Webcrawler use the contents of the Web page description "metatag" if an "invisible" description is read by the search engine but not displayed by your browser. If the description metatag is missing, the first few lines of text on the page are used. For a well-designed page, this is often sufficient. Finally, Excite and Lycos use proprietary methods to extract the concept of a page, assembling dominant sentences as a description.
- *Relevance rating.* Unless a relevance rating is in the high 90s, you most likely should ignore it (the rating, not the result) because what is relevant to one search engine often has more or less relevance to another, based on how the search software was designed and on how the search engine ranks relevant Web sites. Some search engines generate revenue by charging companies a fee to appear prominently in an Internet search. To satisfy yourself that this is true, you should try the same search with each of the major search engines and then com-

pare how closely their relevance rankings match up. Sometimes they do, other times, they do not.

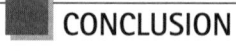 ## CONCLUSION

By defining your search, you will eliminate much of the "noise" you might get with a slot-machine approach. You will find selecting the appropriate tool for each type of search to be easier. And most importantly, you will become an expert in interpreting your results before you spend time examining Web pages that may or may not be of any interest to you. Additionally, in judging whether the information is applicable and credible, Internet users may rely on a number of Internet guides or portals that review and rate Web sites to provide health information. Theoretically, by relying on these ratings, users can identify valuable information more easily. However, if the instruments used to produce the ratings are flawed (for example, if they are produced to sell specific products or if they do not have any discriminative power), they may mislead or misinform health care providers or consumers. (See Chapter 4 for more information on evaluating Web sites.)

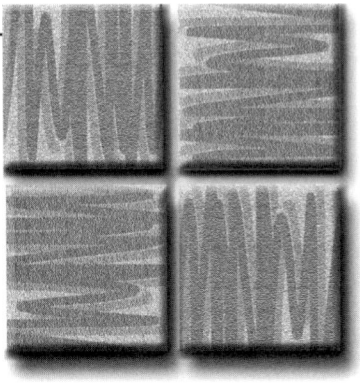

# Searching the Biomedical Literature for Complementary and Alternative Medicine Information

**Chapter Highlights**
Introduction
Strategies for Conducting Searches
Specific Resources Within Complementary
    and Alternative Medicine
Searching PubMed and CAM on PubMed
Using the Cochrane Library
Using the Ovid Collection

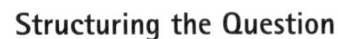

## INTRODUCTION

This chapter will serve as a tutorial for biomedical research-related information on complementary and alternative medicine (CAM). It will start with tools and techniques for defining and conducting searches to answer specific questions concerning CAM and then profile resources that provide the information for answering specific health and medical questions regarding CAM.

## STRATEGIES FOR CONDUCTING SEARCHES

### Structuring the Question

How do you integrate your understanding of the types of tools available in the context of your search strategy, as opposed to using a fomula for finding medical information? From the point of view of a health professional, information searches generally are implemented to find the answer to a question. If the question is clinical, the search has an added urgency. In all cases, your search will be enhanced by knowing the capacity of various search engines and their nuances. Search strategy involves matching your question to the best information resources and then tailoring the search to resources that provide quality content in complementary and alternative medicine. Developing a strategy also entails knowledge of a range of databases. This stage of your search involves critical appraisal:

- What strategy should you use to obtain the best information?
- Where is that information located?

1. **You should define what you are searching for in the clearest possible terms.** More than 350 CAM modalities, 230,000 citations in MEDLINE, and more than 500,000 entries exist on the Internet under "alternative medicine." Consequently, being as precise as possible in your choice of search engines, search strategies, and keywords is important.

2. **How critical is timeliness to your search?** The importance of timely information may be an issue, depending on your need. If you are looking for (clinical) information on a new product or therapy, you will want to broaden your search. Your search may include updates on adverse effects, databases on interactions, recent clinical trials, and even current reporting found in Web archives of the federal government and newspapers such as the *New York Times.* An inevitable time lag in the peer-reviewed medical literature exists because reviewing is tied to the publication process. You should remind yourself that most information in medical journals is at least a year old. An unavoidable time lag occurs from the time the research is completed to the actual publication date.

3. **What type of information are you seeking: efficacy, safety, or quality?** The type of information you seek also will influence how you conduct your search.

4. **What are the optimal sources for information on efficacy?** Efficacy information is based on research in the peer-reviewed literature, reflected in the results of randomized controlled trials and clinical trials.

5. **What are the most effective strategies to obtain information on safety issues?** The following sources are not necessarily different from those on efficacy, but the search strategies differ. You will want to broaden your review to include more resources than simply clinical and controlled trials. For safety information, reporting mechanisms are faster than waiting for published literature from a research trial. This raises the question of who else is monitoring particular issues besides the research community. You do not want to learn 1 year later that a clinical trial was stopped because of a finding of adverse effects or some other concern.

   The scope of your search should include various types of reports, including safety reports and reports in government databases. Target the keywords in your search strategy, using terms such as *safety, adverse effects, contraindications,* and others to capture this topic in the literature. Safety queries have a sense of ur-

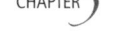

gency, and seeking out resources that include up-to-date information is important. The following Web sites and strategies are suggested:

- The Food and Drug Administration (FDA): **<http://www.fda.gov/>**
- The Centers for Disease Control and Prevention (CDC): **<http://www.cdc.gov/>**
- Watchdog reporting Web sites such as Quack Watch: **<http://www.quackwatch. com/>**
- PubMed: **<http://www.ncbi.nlm.nih.gov>.** You can search PubMed using an advanced search (also described as a Boolean search), for example: "generic or Latin name of product" AND "safety" or "generic or Latin name of product" AND "adverse effects"
- Healthfinder: **<http://www.healthfinder.gov/>.** You can run a keyword search in the health databases of the U.S. government, accessed through Healthfinder.
- *New York Times:* **<http://www.nytimes.com/>.** You can perform an advanced search in the *New York Times* Online Archives.
- American Botanical Council: **<http://www.herbalgram.org/>.** You can access databases on interactions and adverse effects on the site of the American Botanical Council, which includes information based on Commission E, established in 1972 by the German government to evaluate the safety/efficacy of over 300 herbs and herb combinations sold in Germany.
- Medscape: **<http://www.medscape.com/>.** Sites such as Medscape provide topic content, which frequently can be searched by keyword.

6.  **What are the best resources for information about quality?**
    The question of quality usually refers to the content of a botanical or nutraceutical product and tends to involve more subtle issues. In terms of quality issues, multiple resources and multiple databases will be posted across a time continuum. A search strategy involves exploring timely information (most likely from several sites) to access recent periodicals, monographs, reports, Web sites, and the literature. Again, resources extend beyond the peer-reviewed journals. The strategy may involve searching not only MEDLINE, but even new sites such as the *New York Times* Online Archives. You should enter keywords, including the name of the specific botanical or nutraceutical product, paired with terms such as *testing, evaluation, adulteration,* and *purity.* This evaluation involves key questions:

- What does the literature indicate about the effectiveness of this product?
- What should be in the product, based on efficacy reports?
- What is the optimal clinical dose?
- What is the dosage for individuals of different ages, weights, or metabolic types?
- Is the active constituent in a form shown to be clinically effective?
- In the product you are evaluating, is the active herbal constituent or nutrient at the level indicated on the label?

In this search, the overall goal is to be optimally sensitive to the topic, using terminology that will capture as much of the information you are seeking as possible. You also should be precise, so that you are limiting that information to the area you want. If the search is not sensitive enough, information overload is likely to occur.

## Resources for Getting an Overview of the Literature

In creating a hierarchy of medical information, potentially the most fruitful resources to use in the first stage of a search are those that provide an overview—reviews, meta-analyses, and large-scale randomized, controlled trials. In the fields of CAM, major resources that provide reviews include the following:

- CAM on PubMed <http://www.nlm.nih.gov/nccam/camonpubmed.html>
- The Cochrane Library <http://www.update-software.com/cochrane/>
- The Ovid Online Digital Collection <http://www.ovid.com>
- Bandolier, University of Oxford <http://www.jr2.ox.ac.uk/bandolier/kb.html>
- OMNI: Organized Medical Networked Information, UK <http://www.omni.ac.uk/>
- MD Consult <http://www.mdconsult.com/>

When you are not sure what you are looking for (as often seems the case) and you desire a broad overview of an area within complementary medicine or a review of recent articles and trends in CAM, beginning with a database such as MEDLINE/PubMed is better. This particular database is broad and allows you to develop queries to isolate information. This resource is provided at no charge by the National Library of Medicine of the National Institutes of Health (NIH). (MEDLINE/PubMed will not always include a subset of the best literature. Despite the massive size of this collection, some resources are omitted, such as many non-English language publications.) MEDLINE encompasses more than 11 million entries, so it still provides a well-indexed, broad overview that can be applied in your search for information.

In addition to the Cochrane Library and the Ovid evidence-based medicine (EBM) collections, important sources of synthesized informatiom in CAM include Bandolier <http://www.jr2.ox.ac.uk/bandolier/>, of the University of Oxford, which provides an evidence-based synthesis of medical information available online at no charge. OMNI <http://omni.ac.uk/> has collected sources of synthesized reviews on topics that include complementary and alternative medicine. MD Consult <http://www.mdconsult.com/> provides full text of CAM books and medical information texts for a fee.

## SPECIFIC RESOURCES WITHIN COMPLEMENTARY AND ALTERNATIVE MEDICINE

Collections of information focused on specific topics within CAM are now available and are updated on a continual basis. Table 3-1 lists quality information resources.

### Databases and Resources

Depending on your question, you will want to tailor your searches to various databases. For example, some databases are specific to herbals and herbal products, various types of publications such as monographs, or content focused on safety or efficacy. Your search will be defined by the type of information you are seeking and how broad a net you wish to cast. The concept of a net is a useful metaphor in describing search strategies. If you are fishing with a net, you can cast a wide net and catch every-

<table>

|  | | |
|---|---|---|
</table>

### TABLE 3-1 Collections of Information on Complementary and Alternative Medicine

| DATABASE | ACCESS | URL |
|---|---|---|
| **Bandolier**<br>*Complementary Medicine Summaries*<br>Bandolier is a print and Internet journal about health care, using evidence-based medicine techniques to provide advice about particular treatments or diseases for health care professionals and consumers. The content is tertiary publishing, distilling the information from (secondary) reviews of (primary) trials and making it comprehensible. Bandolier contains more than 75 summaries on the effectiveness of complementary therapies. | Free | http://www.jr2.ox.ac.uk/ bandolier/booth/booths/ altmed.html |
| **CAM on PubMed**<br>CAM on PubMed was developed jointly by the National Library of Medicine (NLM) and NCCAM to help persons search easily for journal articles related to a variety of CAM therapies, approaches, and systems. CAM on PubMed contains 220,000 citations, has links to full text, and allows searchers to limit retrievals by publication type. To search, go to the subsets menu and select "Complementary Medicine." | Free | http://www.ncbi.nlm.nih. gov/entrez/query.fcgi? CMD=Limits&DB= PubMed |
| **CISCOM**<br>The Centralized Information Service for Complementary Medicine (CISCOM) of the Research Council for Complementary Medicine, United Kingdom, contains 4000 randomized trials and more than 60,000 citations and abstracts covering and arranged by the major complementary therapies including acupuncture, aromatherapy, healing, hypnotherapy, chiropractic, homeopathy, and manipulation. | Fee to access | http://www.rccm.org.uk/ cisc.htm |
| **Cochrane Complementary Medicine Field Registry**<br>*Complementary Medicine Field*<br>To meet the growing need for evidence-based complementary medicine, the Complementary Medicine Field promotes and facilitates the production and collection of systematic reviews in complementary medicine and continually maintains and updates a registry of randomized controlled trials. The registry is located at the University of Maryland Complementary Medicine Program (CMP). | Free | http://www.compmed. umm.edu/cochrane/ index.html |

*Continued*

| DATABASE | ACCESS | URL |
|---|---|---|
| **Cochrane Library**<br>*Cochrane Collaboration*<br>The Cochrane Library is an electronic publication produced by the Cochrane Collaboration to supply high-quality evidence to inform persons providing and receiving care and those responsible for research, teaching, funding, and administration. The database is published quarterly on CD-ROM and the Internet and is distributed by subscription. The database contains more than 5600 reports of randomized controlled trials and more than 83 systematic reviews in complementary medicine. | Fee to access | http://www.cochrane-library.com/clibhome/clib.htm |
| **HerbMed**<br>HerbMed is an herbal database that provides hyperlinked access to the scientific data underlying the use of herbs for health and is an evidence-based information resource for professionals, researchers, and the general public. HerbMed contains 125 evidence-based reviews of herbal therapies. | Free | http://www.herbmed.org/ |
| **Ovid Best Evidence Collection**<br>More than 90 journals on internal medicine and other specialties such as family practice, pediatrics, obstetrics, psychiatry, gynecology, and surgery are scanned, and only those articles that meet strict selection criteria for study design are selected for review. The articles are summarized in a structured abstract, with expert commentary. The collection can be searched separately but also is available as a limit (EBM reviews) from MEDLINE. The collection contains more than 1500 full-text reports on complementary medicine. | Fee to access | http://www.ovid.com |
| **POEMs: Patient Oriented Evidence That Matters**<br>*Journal of Family Practice*<br>POEMs features reviews of more than 90 journals and identifies the eight articles most important for primary care clinicians to read. POEMs contains coverage of complementary therapies. | Free | http://www.infopoems.com/ |
| **SUMSearch**<br>*University of Texas Health Science Center*<br>SUMSearch is a unique method of searching for medical evidence by using the Internet. SUMSearch combines metasearching and contingency searching to automate searching for medical evidence. SUMSearch covers complementary therapies. | Free | http://www.uthscsa.edu/ |

| TABLE 3-1 Collections of Information on Complementary and Alternative Medicine—cont'd | | |
| --- | --- | --- |
| DATABASE | ACCESS | URL |
| **TRIP Database** | Free | http://www.tripdatabase. |
| *National Health Service, United Kingdom* | | com/ |
| The TRIP Database searches 58 sites of high-quality medical information and gives direct, hyperlinked access to the largest collection of evidence-based material on the Web, as well as articles from premier online journals such as the *British Medical Journal, Journal of the American Medical Association,* and *New England Journal of Medicine.* The database contains evidence-based information on complementary and alternative therapies. | | |
| **University of Maryland Complementary Medicine Program Databases** | Free | http://www.compmed. umm.edu/ |
| This program facilitates systematic literature reviews and evaluation. Other databases include the Arthritis and Complementary and Alternative Medicine Database (ARCAM) and the Complementary and Alternative Medicine and Pain Database (CAMPAIN). | | |

thing. In searches for information on CAM, the sensitivity of your search is also likely to be important (Table 3-2).

## The Story of the Fisherman and His Net

The story of the fisherman and his net (Hans Peter Duer Lecture, Johns Hopkins University, 1999) can be used as a metaphor for searching the biomedical literature for CAM. When the fisherman was asked to describe the fish in the sea, he replied, "All fish are 2 inches or bigger." He then went on to describe the fish in detail. When the listener looked at the fisherman's net, he observed that the holes in his net were 2 inches wide. When he asked the fisherman whether any fish were smaller than 2 inches, the fisherman responded, "Of course not." The point of the story is this: How you define your search and the sensitivity of your strategies will determine what you capture. To optimize your strategy, you should consider the following:

- You should define in the clearest terms what you are seeking.
- You should know where to find the information.
- You should have criteria for evaluating the content once you have found the information.

*Text continued on p. 40*

## TABLE 3-2 Databases and Resources Specific to Complementary and Alternative Medicine

| DATABASE | ACCESS | URL |
|---|---|---|
| **ACUBASE**<br>Published by the Bibliothéque Universitatire de Médicine de Nîmes, this database contains more than 11,000 French and English references and full-text articles dedicated specifically to the discipline of acupuncture. The database also includes conference proceedings. | Fee to access | http://www.trigram.com/default.htm |
| **AGRICultural OnLine Access (AGRICOLA)**<br>This bibliographic database of citations to the agricultural literature was created by the National Agricultural Library and its cooperators and includes citations for herbs and medicinal plants and includes references from HerbalGram of the Herb Research Foundation. | Free | http://www.nal.usda.gov/ag98/ |
| **Allied and Complementary Medicine (AMED)**<br>AMED is a unique database produced by the Health Care Information Service of the British Library and includes resources for complementary medicine, palliative care, and several professions allied with medicine. AMED is available in a variety of formats, from print to online. | Fee to access | http://www.bl.uk/ |
| **AltHealthWatch**<br>*EBSCO Information Services*<br>This is a Web-based, full-text database of periodicals, peer-reviewed journals, academic and professional publications, magazines, consumer newsletters and newspapers. | Fee to access | http://www.epnet.com/eptech/ |
| **ClinicalTrials.gov**<br>This site provides current information on disease treatment at particular institutions or by a disease, drug, modality, therapy, or procedure. The site contains complementary and alternative medicine therapies (search by words: "alternative" [medicine or therapy] or "complementary" [medicine or therapy], by particular modality [acupuncture], or by a particular substance [ginko or shark cartilage]). | Free | http://clinicaltrials.gov/ |
| **Cumulative Index to Nursing and Allied Health (CINAHL)**<br>CINAHL indexes alternative medicine journals. | Fee to access | http://www.cinahl.com/ |

## TABLE 3-2 Databases and Resources Specific to Complementary and Alternative Medicine—cont'd

| DATABASE | ACCESS | URL |
|---|---|---|
| **Datadiwan**<br>Datadiwan provides access to information on holistic medicine and frontier sciences. Second, Datadiwan is a scientific discussion forum in which interested parties can discuss scientific topics with other like-minded persons around the world. Third, Datadiwan is a network that links research institutions and organizations worldwide. Most of the literature is in German. | Free | http://www.datadiwan.de/index_e.htm |
| **Dr. Duke's Phytochemical and Ethnobotanical Databases**<br>*Agricultural Research Service, U.S. Department of Agriculture (ARS, USDA)*<br>The ARS, USDA, databases can be searched by chemical, specific activity, or ethnobotanical usage. | Free | http://www.ars-grin.gov/duke/index/html |
| **EMBASE**<br>This international database contains citations covering the biomedical, pharmacological, and drug literature. | Fee to access | http://www.embase.com/ |
| **EthnobotDB (Plant Uses Worldwide)**<br>James A. Duke and Stephen M. Beckstrom-Sternberg, of the National Germplasm Resources Laboratory (NGRL), ARS, USDA, built this database, which contains 80,000 records of plant uses. | Free | http://www.ars-grin.gov/duke/index/html |
| **HerbMed**<br>This herbal database provides hyperlinked access to the scientific data underlying the use of herbs for health and is an evidence-based information resource for professionals, researchers, and general public. The database is a project of the Alternative Medicine Foundation. | Free | http://www.herbmed.org/ |
| **Hom-Inform Database**<br>This database of indexed literature references in homeopathy is produced by the British Homeopathic Library at Glasgow Homeopathic Hospital and is searchable online. | Free | http://hominform.soutron.com/ |

*Continued*

**TABLE 3-2** Databases and Resources Specific to Complementary and Alternative Medicine—cont'd

| DATABASE | ACCESS | URL |
|---|---|---|
| International Bibliographic Information on Dietary Supplements (IBIDS)<br>This database is produced by the Office of Dietary Supplements, NIH, along with the Food and Nutrition Information Center, National Agricultural Library, USDA. IBIDS contains bibliographic records, including abstracts published in international scientific journals on the topic of dietary supplements, including vitamins, minerals, and herbal and botanical supplements. The general public, scientists, researchers, and others can search the database using keywords to obtain the citations of research journal articles. | Free | http://ods.od.nih.gov/databases/ibids.html |
| Manual, Alternative and Natural Therapy (MANTIS) Database (formerly CHIROLARS)<br>Coverage for health care disciplines not represented significantly in the major biomedical databases. References are from more than 1000 journals, with preference given to peer-reviewed journals. MANTIS includes health promotion and prevention, acupuncture, allopathic medicine, alternative medicine, chiropractic, herbal medicine, homeopathy, naturopathy, osteopathic medicine, physical therapy, and Chinese medicine. | Fee to access | http://www.healthindex.com |
| Medicinal Plants of Native America Database (MPNADB)<br>This database "contains 17,634 items representing the medicinal uses of 2,147 species from 760 genera and 142 families by 123 different native American groups—was built over a period of about 10 years with support from the National Endowment for the Humanities, the National Science Foundation, and the University of Michigan-Dearborn." | Free | http://www.umd.umich.edu/cgi-bin/herb |
| MEDLINE/PubMed<br>The best interface is PubMed from the NLM, Bethesda, Maryland. The MEDLINE database supports the teachings and research of the current medical system in the United States. The database contains 11 million citations and includes the complementary medicine subset CAM on PubMed. | Free | http://www.ncbi.nlm.nih.gov/entrez/<br>http://www.nlm.nih.gov/nccam/camonpubmed.html |

**TABLE 3-2** Databases and Resources Specific to Complementary and Alternative Medicine—cont'd

| DATABASE | ACCESS | URL |
|---|---|---|
| **MICROMEDEX Complementary & Alternative Medicine (CAM) Series**<br>The Complementary & Alternative Medicine Series from MICROMEDEX is a comprehensive, clinically focused reference tool based on a thorough compilation of scientific literature. Monographs in the series present data on administration, dosing, warnings, precautions, contraindications, and interactions. | Fee to access | http://www.micromedex.com/products/healthcare/cam/si-8753.pdf |
| **MICROMEDEX Herbal & Alternative Remedies**<br>*American Academy of Family Physicians,*<br>*familydoctor.org*<br>This database of alternative medicines has an alphabetically arranged index and allows searches by name. Information is provided by AltCareDex and is produced by MICROMEDEX Thomson Healthcare products. | Fee to access | http://www.familydoctor.org/cgi-bin/altcaredex_search |
| **National Center for Complementary and Alternative Medicine**<br>CAM databases include CAM on PubMed. Bibliographic citations are obtained from the NLM PubMed (MEDLINE) database that uses a feature to locate citations with a predetermined CAM search criteria. | Free | http://www.nlm.nih.gov/nccam/camonpubmed.html |
| **Native American Ethnobotany Database**<br>Dan Moerman, professor of anthropology at the University of Michigan-Dearborn, describes the database as "foods, drugs, dyes, fibers and other uses of plants (a total of over 47,000 items). This represents uses by 291 Native American groups of 3,895 species from 243 different plant families." | Free | http://www.umd.umich.edu/cgi-bin/herb |
| **Natural Medical Protocols for Doctors**<br>This Web-accessible fee-based service "includes current research data and treatment protocols for most common medical conditions and cross-linked reference material about vitamins, minerals, herbs, homeopathy and other supplements and therapies. The information was gathered and organized by a consortium of doctors from various branches of medicine. This includes MDs (conventional medical doctors), NDs (naturopathic doctors), acupuncturists and PhDs of various kinds. The data compiled here was taken from research journals (through 2000) and medical books and the reference citations are included." | Fee to access | http://www.natmedpro.com/ |

*Continued*

**TABLE 3-2** Databases and Resources Specific to Complementary and Alternative Medicine—cont'd

| DATABASE | ACCESS | URL |
|---|---|---|
| **Natural Medicines Comprehensive Database** *Pharmacist's Letter/Prescriber's Letter* This database provides clinical data on the natural medicines, herbal medicines, and dietary supplements used in the Western world and is compiled by pharmacists and physicians. | Fee to access | http://www. naturaldatabase.com/ |
| **Natural Products ALERT (NAPRALERT)** *STN International* This database contains bibliographic and factual data on natural products, including information on the pharmacology, biological activity, taxonomic distribution, ethnomedicine, and chemistry of plant, microbial, and animal (including marine) extracts. In addition, the file contains data on the chemistry and pharmacology of secondary metabolites that are derived from natural sources and that have known structures. The NAPRALERT file contains more than 100,000 records from 1650 to the present. About 50% of the file is from systematic survey of the literature from 1975 to the present. The remaining records were obtained by selective retrospective indexing dating back to 1650. | Fee to access | http://info.cas.org/ ONLINE/DBSS/ napralertss.html |
| **Nutritionals Adverse Event Monitoring System** *U.S. FDA, Center for Food Safety & Applied Nutrition, Office of Special Nutritionals* This database of adverse effects is compiled from the use of special nutritional products—dietary supplements, infant formulas, and medical foods—as reported by health professionals and consumers. | Free | http://www.cfsan.fda.gov/ |
| **Patent Database** *U.S. Patent and Trademark Office* This tool locates registered patents in complementary and alternative medicine. | Free | http://www.uspto.gov/ patft/index.html |

**TABLE 3-2** Databases and Resources Specific to Complementary and Alternative Medicine—cont'd

| DATABASE | ACCESS | URL |
|---|---|---|
| **PhytoNet**<br>*Centre for Complementary Health Studies, University of Exeter*<br>PhytoNet is a "resource for those involved in the development, manufacture, regulation and surveillance of phytomedicines and herbal drugs" and contains information from the European Scientific Co-operative on Phytotherapy (ESCOP), forms to submit adverse effects of herbal medicines, and European standards for safe use of phytomedicines. | Free | http://www.escop.com/ phytonet.htm |
| **Phytotherapies.org Monograph Database**<br>This database is a free service to individuals registering with the site and is "sponsored by Herbworx Corporation, an Australian company dedicated to ensuring that practitioners are supplied not only with high quality herbal medicine, but also clinically relevant, scientifically validated technical information, and Phytomedicine manufacturer quality herbal extracts for practitioners." Even though the service is commercial, the herbal monograph database contains indications, actions, constituents, studies, and articles. | Free | http://www.phytotherapies. org/ |
| **Poisonous Plant Database**<br>*U.S. FDA, Center for Food Safety & Applied Nutrition, Office of Plant and Dairy Foods and Beverages*<br>The Poisonous Plant Database is a set of working files of scientific information about the animal and human toxicology of vascular plants of the world. | Free | http://vm.cfsan.fda.gov/~ djw/readme.html |
| **PsychInfo**<br>*American Psychological Association*<br>PsychInfo is a source for mind-body and other complementary and alternative therapies used in mental disorders, stress reduction, or psychological and behavioral processes and neuroimmunology. | Fee to access | http://www.apa.org/ psycinfo/ |

##  SEARCHING PUBMED AND CAM ON PUBMED

### What PubMed Is

PubMed is an extensive database of the National Library of Medicine. PubMed and Grateful Med are two interfaces for searching the MEDLINE database. The PubMed interface includes MEDLINE and about 40 other databases such as molecular biology databases.

### How to Access PubMed

PubMed, MEDLINE, and CAM on PubMed are provided by the National Center for Biotechnology Information (NCBI) at <**http://www.ncbi.nih.gov/**>.

### What PubMed Provides

MEDLINE and its related databases contain summaries (citations) of journal articles in the peer-reviewed medical literature, cataloging millions of clinical studies and review articles from the world literature. MEDLINE contains entries totaling more than 11 million citations, including clinical studies, systematic reviews, meta-analyses, and even letters to the editor, all indexed from about 4000 journals, with more than 400,000 new articles added annually. In PubMed, you can browse specific themes using keywords, which provides a search of more than 11 million journals in a matter of seconds. PubMed is user-friendly: its technology allows the end-user to go beyond the medical terminology.

### Components of PubMed

PubMed is the more recent interface developed for searching MEDLINE, accessed from the home page of NCBI. PubMed provides searches of MEDLINE that are faster, more comprehensive, and more flexible than earlier interfaces. Grateful Med is the original software used to access MEDLINE, until PubMed was brought online in 1996.

### How PubMed Works

The system is designed around complex algorithms and mapping functions. Medical subject headings (MeSH) that have been defined from the medical literature are stored in a medical thesaurus; these terms define and speed up the search. By determining the precise terms needed for your search, you can maximize and focus the information you capture. An online thesaurus and medical dictionary are available along with a tutorial that describes how to use the system.

### Additional Features of PubMed

Some of the journal articles cited on MEDLINE include links to full text. Where available, the link will be indicated by a logo to the right of the article title. This link usually takes you to the full-text article on the Web site of the publisher if available or to the journal where you can order the article (Fig. 3-1). In some cases, such as with American Medical Association journals, the linked text can be accessed only by mem-

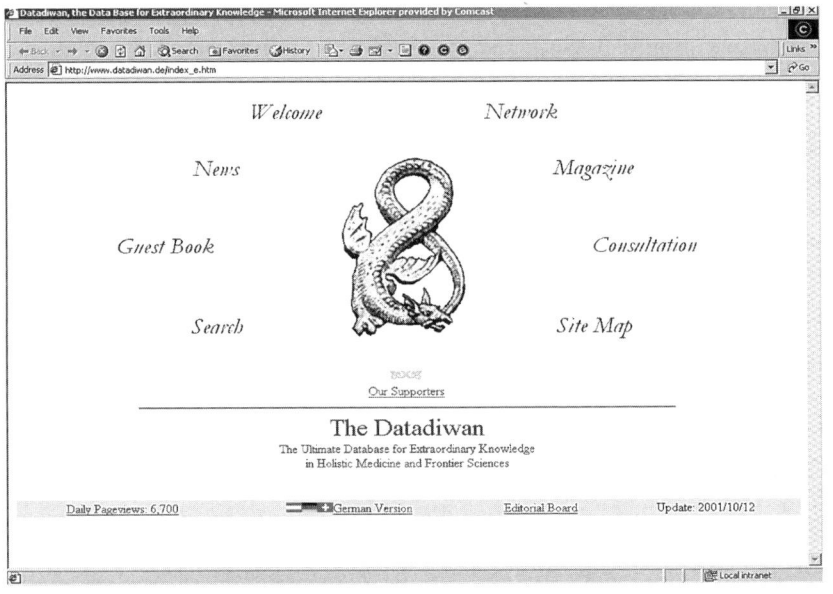

FIG. 3-1   ▪   The home page of Datadiwan, one possible link from a search of CAM literature on PubMed.

bers or subscribers. However, certain journals are still available to all visitors, such as those of the *British Medical Journal* at **<http://www.bmj.com/>**.

## Information Available on CAM on PubMed

The largest and best-known complementary medicine database is CAM on PubMed, essentially a subset of PubMed. This CAM database now includes more than 220,000 citations specifically on complementary medicine that can be accessed using keywords and topics relevant to CAM. Web users now also have the option of limiting PubMed searches to complementary medicine. The collection was one of the first U.S.-based government-sponsored initiatives in collecting the CAM literature. Before this database became available on PubMed, it was available as a free-standing collection on the Web site of NCCAM **<http://www.nccam.nih.gov/>**.

## Search Strategies

Originally the use of keywords was essential to search MEDLINE. These words and phrases were organized and cataloged in a metathesauras of medical subject (MeSH) headings. Understanding the way a particular term is mapped provides insight into useful search strategies, particularly if you are seeking difficult-to-find material. In earlier versions of MEDLINE software, unless the precise MeSH term was used, the search would not yield any relevant results. For example, a search of Vitamin C would yield no results, whereas a search of ascorbic acid produced more than 20,000 citations.

Although the metathesaurus of PubMed seems to be mapped to many more terms, beginning your search by checking the MeSHs to focus your topic is still helpful.

### Limitations of PubMed

About 50,000 of the 220,000 citations included in the CAM on PubMed database are located by just searching under the MeSH "alternative medicine." Additionally, if you are looking for clinical trials, searching other collections is best; for example, the Cochrane Library or the Complementary Medicine Field Registry, which has collected more than 6000 clinical trials in the CAM literature.

### Benefits of PubMed

MEDLINE is an exceptional resource available at no cost that provides rapid, comprehensive searches of the literature, summarized findings, and in some cases, links to full text.

 ## USING THE COCHRANE LIBRARY

### What the Library Is

The Cochrane Collaboration is an international consortium: 11 centers are located primarily in academic medical centers worldwide. The Cochrane Library Controlled Trials Registry contains research on more than 300,000 controlled clinical studies. The Cochrane Collection also includes 1000 meta-analyses, or systematic reviews that are developed from the medical literature and intended to serve the needs of physicians, researchers, policy makers, consumers, and other stakeholders.

Cochrane fields and networks are groups that focus on dimensions of health care other than specific diagnoses, such as the setting of care (for example, primary care), the type of consumer (for example, older people), the type of provider (for example, nurses), or the type of intervention (for example, physical therapy).

### How to Access the Library

The Cochrane Library is published quarterly on CD-ROM and the Internet <http://www.update-software.com/cochrane/cochrane-frame.html> and is distributed by subscription. Additionally, ordering and price information for the CD-ROM can be obtained by calling Update Software in Vista, California, at (760) 631-5844.

### What the Library Provides

Cochrane review groups, fields, and networks develop their own registries of clinical trials, which they maintain and update by consistently collecting information from the world literature. The mission of the collaboration is to gather as much information as possible, primarily clinical controlled trials and randomized controlled trials, from all the fields of medicine, organize it within a single system, and make the information available to researchers and clinicians.

## Components of the Library

Several databases are included in the Cochrane Library:

- The Cochrane Database of Systematic Reviews contains Cochrane reviews.
- The Cochrane Controlled Trials Register is a bibliographic database of controlled trials.
- The Database of Abstracts of Reviews of Effectiveness (DARE) includes structured abstracts of systematic reviews that have been appraised critically by reviewers at the National Health Service Center, United Kingdom.

## Systematic Reviews in the Library

To perform a review within the Cochrane Collaboration, an evaluation protocol must be posted electronically, identifying the topic area, intentions, search strategy, databases to be searched, references, and reviewers. A collection of full-text articles is amassed, and the analysis is executed over a period of about 6 months. The reviews are performed to a high standard, using exhaustive searches that include non-English language studies while controlling for publication bias and study quality. Once completed, the review is published electronically by the Cochrane Collaboration with a period for comment, which provides peer review.

As such, the Cochrane systematic reviews evaluate all the randomized controlled trials in a particular field, rating each study and comparing the data, combining the results wherever possible; as a result, rather than having a single study with a small sample size and little statistical power, more than one study sample can be combined. In doing so, systematic reviews provide a means of cohering what sometimes can be contradictory information, summarizing the state of the science, and determining the clinical effectiveness of various methods of treatment, including complementary therapies.

## Information Available on Complementary and Alternative Medicine

The Cochrane Library is perhaps one of the best single sources for information on complementary therapies and EBM. The Complementary Medicine Field, working within the Cochrane Collaboration, specifically focuses on complementary medicine. Typically, Cochrane fields are related to a general crosscutting area, such as primary care. Other centers are comparable to the NIH, with a focus on multiple related topics such as musculoskeletal disorders or diabetes and digestive diseases. The Complementary Medicine Field has established its own registry, conducts reviews, and tracks other Cochrane reviews that meet the defining guidelines for complementary medicine. The collection currently contains 90 systematic reviews in Complememtary Medicine, with an additional 53 reviews now in progress. Physicians, through subscription to the Cochrane Library, can obtain evidence-based information on complementary therapies, which reflects clinical outcomes on effectiveness and safety of CAM interventions.

### Fees of the Library

The publications of the Cochrane Library are available for a fee: on CD-ROM for about $200 per year and online by subscription.

## Benefits of the Library

The Cochrane Library is updated and amended as new evidence becomes available and errors are identified; electronic media offer obvious advantages for disseminating and interrogating its contents. The Cochrane Library is disseminated on CD-ROM and on the Internet.

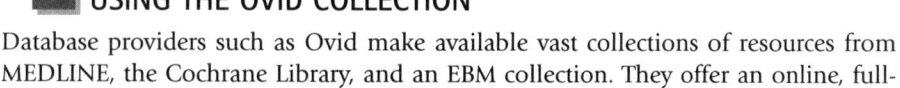 USING THE OVID COLLECTION

Database providers such as Ovid make available vast collections of resources from MEDLINE, the Cochrane Library, and an EBM collection. They offer an online, full-text biomedical collection that includes about 2000 articles on complementary medicine drawn from the medical journals. Ovid also offers MEDLINE and International Pharmaceutical Abstracts. The Ovid interface allows MeSH mapping, journal searching, free text searching, and the ability to perform advanced Boolean searches that include subheadings or qualifiers. Saving searches and re-creating them at a later time is possible as well.

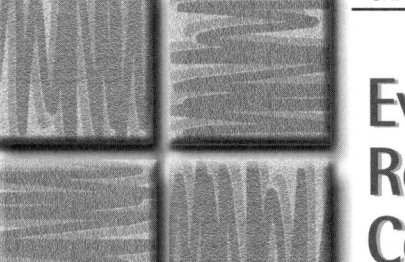

# Evaluating Internet Resources in Complementary and Alternative Medicine

**Chapter Highlights**
Introduction
Issue of Quality
Quality Initiatives for Rating and Evaluating Health
    Sites
Guidelines for Evaluating Web Sites and Managing
    Internet Health Communications
Conclusion

 INTRODUCTION

The goal of this chapter is to discuss standards for medical and CAM information on the Internet and define and describe existing quality initiatives for Internet health care sites and the organizations that post medical and CAM information. The question of quality of information may be the greatest challenge in health information on the Internet. Health care Web sites, now totaling more than 100,000, have rapidly expanded to address the demand for medical information on diseases and other specific conditions. This material, written in the informal language of the Internet, has the potential to empower the public by improving their understanding of health care issues and their own health and by enhancing their ability to participate actively in their own care.[1] In addition, discussion groups and online communities devoted to specific conditions and diseases can publicize local resources and provide valuable emotional and social support.

## ISSUE OF QUALITY

Although immediate access to medical and CAM information has been of great benefit to health care professionals, patients, and consumers, concern is growing that a substantial proportion of Internet-based medical information, and particularly CAM information, is inaccurate, erroneous, misleading, or fraudulent and is thereby a threat to public health.[2-4] Tracking health claims on the Internet is a special focus of the investigative work of the U.S. Federal Trade Commission (FTC). In 1997 the agency began a coordinated effort with the U.S. FDA, Health Canada, and various state attorneys general offices called Operation Cure All. The mission of this operation is "to crack down on companies that use the Internet to prey on the sickest and most vulnerable consumers" by marketing supplements and other products with unsubstantiated health and safety claims. On June 14, 2001, the FTC announced that it and its partner agencies had taken enforcement actions against six companies for fraudulent marketing on the Internet. The products were being marketed to treat or cure cancer, HIV/AIDS (acquired immunodefiency syndrome), arthritis, hepatitis, Alzheimer's disease, diabetes, and other conditions. Specifically, Operation Cure All has taken action on a Web site that was encouraging patients with HIV or AIDS to use St. John's wort as a safe and effective treatment, when in fact the herb is known to interfere with the effectiveness of the AIDS drug indinavir. In a similar enforcement action, a suit was filed against a multilevel marketing company that had claimed the FDA considered its herbal products safe. These products, however, contained comfrey, which is known to pose significant risks to humans, including liver damage.[5]

Although the FTC has the regulatory authority to regulate U.S. prescription drug and medical device advertising on the Internet, an obvious limitation is that the Internet is international, and therefore much of its content is well beyond the reach of the FTC or FDA. Furthermore, in striking down the Computer Decency Act of 1996, U.S. courts have demonstrated a reluctance to support governmental control and cen-

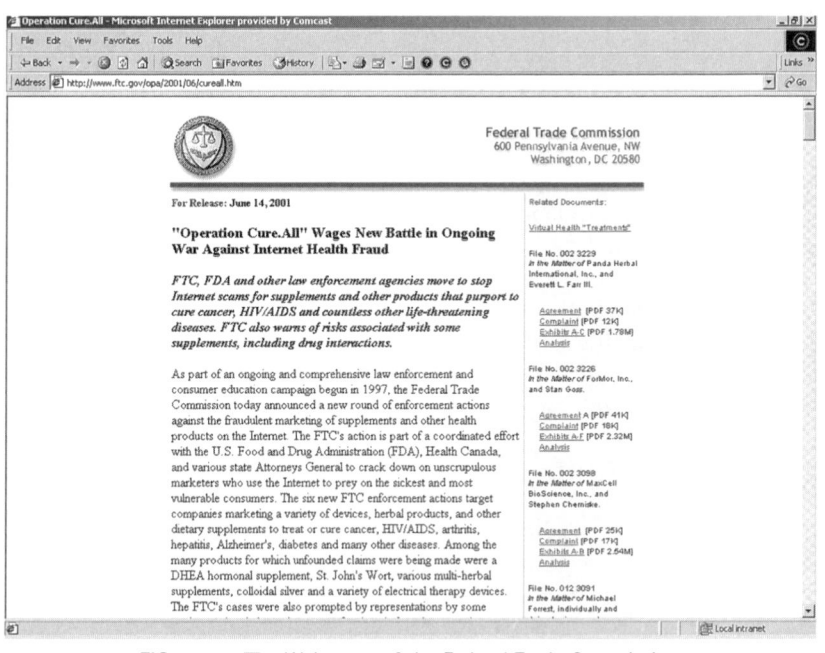

FIG. 4-1 ■ Web page of the Federal Trade Commission.

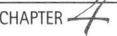

sorship of a medium described as "the most participatory form of mass speech yet developed"[4] (Figs. 4-1 and 4-2).

## QUALITY INITIATIVES FOR RATING AND EVALUATING HEALTH SITES

Medical information that is free from central editorial control is expected to continue to accumulate on the Internet. A few published studies have attempted to characterize the reliability of such information in general terms by investigating its quality regarding specific topics disseminated through discussion groups or on the World Wide Web. For example, Culver, Gerr, and Frumkin[6] studied a discussion group for sufferers of painful hand and arm conditions. In their review of more than 1600 messages, they found that about 90% of the messages providing medical information were authored by persons without professional medical training and that about one third of all medical information provided could best be categorized as "unconventional or CAM." In a broader and more systematic survey of the World Wide Web, Impicciatore and others[7] used search engines to identify parent-oriented Web sites that provided advice for managing childhood fever. Of the 41 Web sites identified at that time, only four adhered closely to published guidelines for home management of childhood fever, and some pages proposed potentially dangerous remedies.

One can argue that the Internet suffers no more from error and inaccuracy than do many traditional informal sources of health care information, including pamphlets

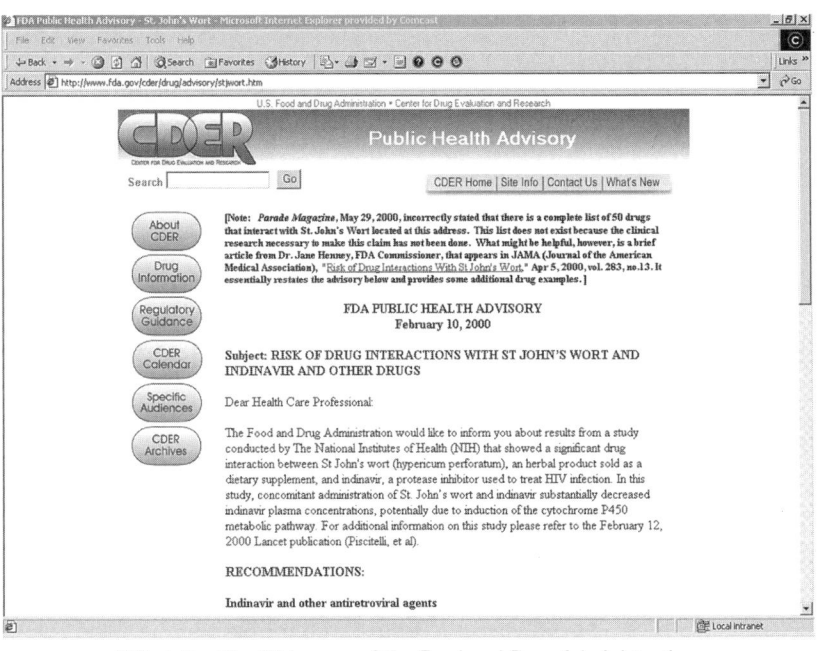

FIG. 4-2 ■ Web page of the Food and Drug Administration.

and popular press articles. However, discerning what constitutes medically authoritative information is difficult, particularly if a site is using official-looking seals and logos.[8] Another concern is that given the nature of the Internet, the potential for harm is enormous because nearly 100 million Americans regularly go online to search for health information.[9,10]

In response to the call for quality, Internet seals of approval, awards, and stamps of approval that rate health information sites have proliferated. However, many of the instruments are developed incompletely and continue to be used by Web sites providing health information on the Internet even after the sponsoring institution that created the instrument no longer exists.[8] Using various strategies to identify these award-like rating instruments, Jadad and Gagliardi[11] performed an exhaustive search of the Internet in 1998. Of the 47 rating instruments identified, only 14 described the criteria used to produce the ratings, and none provided information concerning construct validity. The authors therefore concluded that in general these instruments are developed poorly and are of questionable value. In a follow-up study, Gagliardi and Jadad[8] identified an additional 51 instruments with similar conclusions, bringing the total to 98. Of the 51, only five provided enough information to be evaluated properly.

Other initiatives include a growing number of organizations including government and nonprofit organizations that have developed guidelines and criteria to organize and identify valid health care information on the Internet (Fig. 4-3). The initiatives listed in Table 4-1 are among the best.

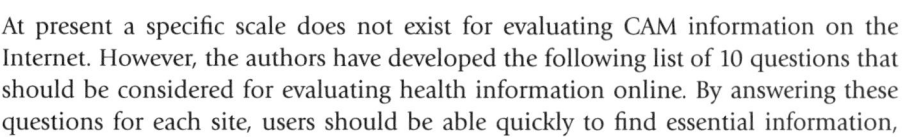

## GUIDELINES FOR EVALUATING WEB SITES AND MANAGING INTERNET HEALTH COMMUNICATIONS

At present a specific scale does not exist for evaluating CAM information on the Internet. However, the authors have developed the following list of 10 questions that should be considered for evaluating health information online. By answering these questions for each site, users should be able quickly to find essential information, evaluate it, and quickly decide whether it is useful.

1. **Who is the originator of the site?**
   Any good health site makes learning who is responsible for the site and its information an easy task. You should not have to be a cyberdetective to figure this out.
2. **What is the purpose of the site?**
   The mission of the site relates to the goals and values of the originator. The purpose of the site should be stated clearly in "About this site" or in a mission statement. Usually a statement is made that the site provides "unbiased and accurate health information."
3. **What is the source of the information?**
   Many of sites essentially recycle information from other Web sites or offline resources. If the Web site lists the source of information, that is obviously of value.

**TABLE 4-1 Health Care Quality Awards, Guides, and Initiatives**

| GUIDE OR CODE | URL | AUDIENCE | MECHANISM | PHILOSOPHY |
|---|---|---|---|---|
| eHealth Code of Ethics | http://www.ihealthcoalition.org/ethics/ethics.html | Consumers | Guide | Code of conduct |
| Hi-Ethics | http://www.hiethics.com | Consumers and member companies | Quality seal | Third-party certification or voluntary compliance with code of conduct |
| MedCERTAIN | http://www.medcertain.org | Consumers | Metatags created by the site provider allow consumers to evaluate content based on tags or rating or trust mark | Voluntary metatags Trust mark Third-party certification |
| American Accreditation HealthCare Commission (URAC) | http://www.urac.org | Providers, consumers, and patients | Directory of approved organizations | Accreditation based on application (fee) |
| Health on the Net (HON) | http://www.hon.ch/ | Consumers | Quality seal | Code of conduct |
| Health Improvement Institute | http://www.hii.org/ | Consumers | Award | Award or code of conduct |
| OMNI | http://omni.ac.uk | Research and academic | Manual filtering | Third-party evaluation based on quality criteria |
| DISCERN | http://www.discern.org.uk | Consumers | Tool-based filtering | Tool-based assessment |
| American Medical Association (AMA) | http://www.ama-assn.org/ama/pub/category/1905.html | AMA site consumers | Self-regulation of own sites | Code of conduct |

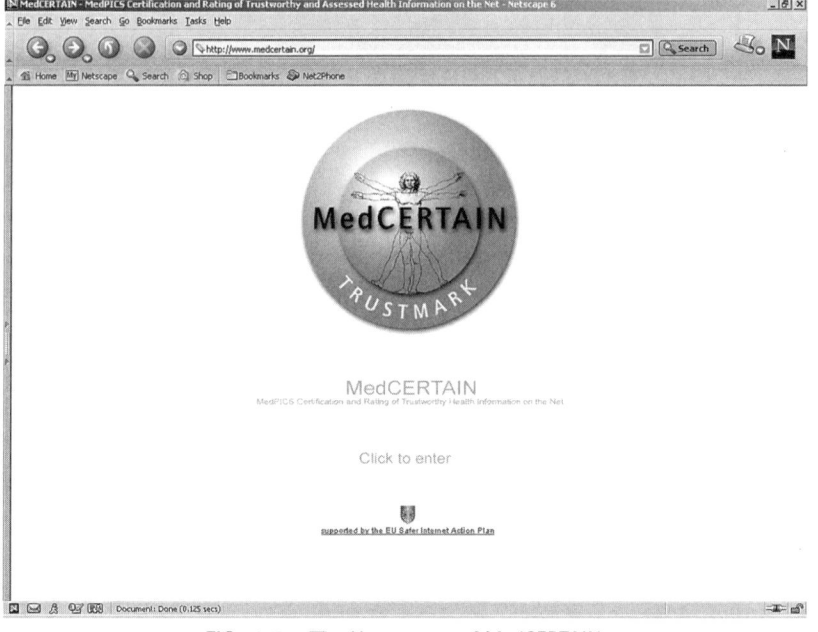

FIG. 4-3 ■ Home page of MedCERTAIN.

4. **What is the basis of the information?**
   What evidence exists to support the information? Are facts and figures from medical research given? Is the information referenced to a journal or consensus statement? Has an expert panel reviewed the evidence? That type of information should be set apart and should be clearly ascertainable.
5. **How is the information selected?**
   The better sites are peer reviewed: their development of content includes a review process by an outside medical board or outside independent agency.
6. **How current is the information?**
   Given the rapid development of information in science and on the Web, updated information and clearly marked pages showing the date of the last update are important factors. Even if the information has not changed, consistent updates indicate a tidy and well-managed site.
7. **Does a policy explain the basis for selecting the links on a site or give some explanation that suggests the relationships?**
   Obviously, advertising is one of the sources of links in e-commerce. If the links are to advertisers, such as pharmaceutical or nutraceutical companies, usually that should be explained. The medical information or content should not be tied directly to an advertisement. If you are reading about kava kava, you should not see a flashing pop-up ad selling Kava Kava.

8. **Who funds the site?**

   The apparent differences between sites are easy to discern: dot-com, dot-org, or dot-gov. Beyond this identification, what is the nature of the site and how does the site generate revenue? Is the site selling advertising or is it sponsored by a manufacturer? Could the source of the funding potentially affect the content? These considerations overlap with those such as the presentation, links, and affiliations of the site.

9. **What information does the site collect?**

   Web sites routinely track visitors and may ask end users to subscribe or become members. Usually this solicitation occurs at no charge, but by it Web sites are able to collect information about users. All sites that register users should tell you exactly what they will and will not do with that information. Many commercial sites sell aggregate data about users to other companies. Such information includes information on gender, the purpose of inquiries (such as a particular condition or disease state), e-mail address, and Zip code. Most importantly, if you enter your Zip code, the Web site operators will know where you live and your gender, and occasionally they will know your birth date if you enter that. A privacy policy must state what the Web site operators are going to do with the information so users are well aware of the risks of giving out medical information over the Internet.

10. **How does the site manage interactions with visitors?**

    How do users and site operators correspond? Does such correspondence occur in a timely way? Do the individuals that correspond with visitors have professional credentials in the areas that they are addressing? In a chat room, who is the moderator and what are that person's credentials? If a discussion area is moderated, who is moderating and why? On many Web sites, the moderators of discussion areas are unpaid, so the level of expertise may be uneven. What are the standards the site uses for recruiting moderators who will interact with patients or consumers on health topics? What is the privacy policy? What is good advice, and what is dangerous advice? In the case of chat rooms, users should always take the time to determine how the online interaction works before becoming participants.

 ## CONCLUSION

For now, what constitutes the gold standard for health information on the Internet is not entirely clear. Standards advocated by Silberg, Lundberg, and Musacchio,[10] such as authorship, attribution, and disclosure, are significant and are identified readily. Measures of scientific quality, accessibility, timeliness, and readability, however, also need to be evaluated but are more difficult to rate reliably. Furthermore, medical information that is free from central editorial control is expected to continue to accumulate on the Internet, and even if validated rating instruments are adopted and in widespread use, they do not relieve health care providers, patients, and consumers of the responsibility to approach Internet health information critically.[12,13]

## References

1. Ferguson T: Health online and the empowered medical consumer, *J Comm J Qual Improv* 23(5):251-257, 1997.
2. Pallen MJ: Medicine and the Internet: dreams, nightmares and reality, *Br J Hosp Med* 56(10):506-509, 1996.
3. Bower H: Internet sees growth of unverified health claims, *BMJ* 313(7054):381, 1996.
4. Sonnenberg FA: Health information on the Internet: opportunities and pitfalls, *Arch Intern Med* 157(2):151-152, 1997.
5. Stickel F, Seitz HK: The efficacy and safety of comfrey, *Public Health Nutr* 3(4A):501-508, 2000.
6. Culver JD, Gerr F, Frumkin H: Medical information on the Internet: a study of an electronic bulletin board, *J Gen Intern Med* 12(8):466-470, 1997.
7. Impicciatore P and others: Reliability of health information for the public on the World Wide Web: systematic survey of advice on managing fever in children at home, *BMJ* 314(7098):1875-1879, 1997.
8. Gagliardi A, Jadad AR: Examination of instruments used to rate quality of health information on the Internet: chronicle of a voyage with an unclear destination, *BMJ* 324(7337):569-573, 2002.
9. Poll H: *www.harrisinteractive.com/harris_poll/index.asp*, 2001.
10. Silberg WM, Lundberg GD, Musacchio RA: Assessing, controlling, and assuring the quality of medical information on the Internet: caveat lector et viewor—let the reader and viewer beware, *JAMA* 277(15):1244-1245, 1997.
11. Jadad AR, Gagliardi A: Rating health information on the Internet: navigating to knowledge or to Babel? *JAMA* 279(8):611-614, 1998.
12. Widman LE, Tong DA: Requests for medical advice from patients and families to health care providers who publish on the World Wide Web, *Arch Intern Med* 157(2):209-212, 1997.
13. Eysenbach G, Kohler C: How do consumers search for and appraise health information on the World Wide Web? Qualitative study using focus groups, usability tests, and in-depth interviews, *BMJ* 324(7337):573-577, 2002:

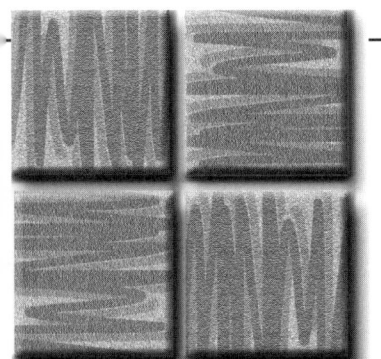

# Complementary and Alternative Medicine Resources by Modality

**Chapter Highlights**
Introduction
Acupuncture
Herbal Medicine
Manual Therapies

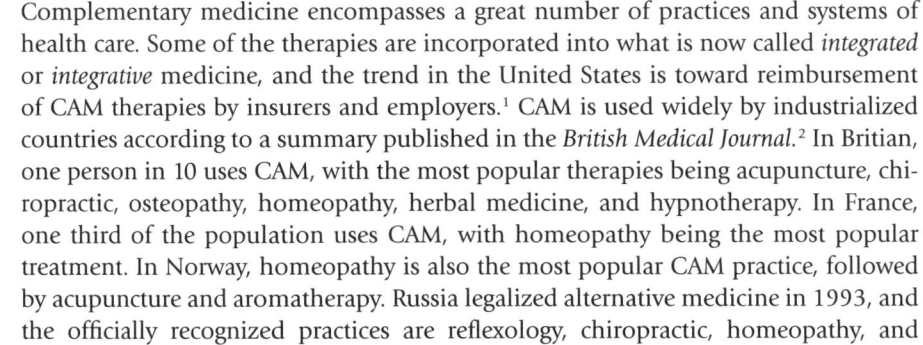

## INTRODUCTION

Complementary medicine encompasses a great number of practices and systems of health care. Some of the therapies are incorporated into what is now called *integrated* or *integrative* medicine, and the trend in the United States is toward reimbursement of CAM therapies by insurers and employers.[1] CAM is used widely by industrialized countries according to a summary published in the *British Medical Journal.*[2] In Britian, one person in 10 uses CAM, with the most popular therapies being acupuncture, chiropractic, osteopathy, homeopathy, herbal medicine, and hypnotherapy. In France, one third of the population uses CAM, with homeopathy being the most popular treatment. In Norway, homeopathy is also the most popular CAM practice, followed by acupuncture and aromatherapy. Russia legalized alternative medicine in 1993, and the officially recognized practices are reflexology, chiropractic, homeopathy, and breathing methods. In Australia, a third of the population regularly visits natural therapists, and two thirds regularly take vitamins and use other natural treatments, the most popular being chiropractic, naturopathy, massage, herbal medicine, and homeopathy. In Japan, two thirds of the population in Tokyo report using CAM treatments. The most popular CAM therapies are herbal medicine, acupuncture, and acupressure (*shiatsu*), and more than 600 herbal medicines are available under the national health insurance system. In Germany and the United Kingdom the national health systems also cover many CAM practices.[3] With increased interest and use worldwide, CAM is one of the fastest growing areas of medicine.

## ACUPUNCTURE

Although acupuncture has been offered in the Asian communities throughout the United States for many generations and in China for thousands of years, only since 1970, following the opening of China to the West, has this system of health care been available to the general U.S. population.

The effects of acupuncture, particularly on pain, can be described within a conventional physiological model. Acupuncture is known to stimulate nerve fibers entering the dorsal horn of the spinal cord. This stimulation can mediate pain impulses carried through connections in the midbrain and inhibit pain impulses at other levels of the spinal cord. This helps explain why acupuncture needles in one part of the body can affect pain sensation in another part. Acupuncture also is known to stimulate the release of endorphins and other neurotransmitters such as serotonin.

### Food and Drug Administration Reclassification Process

In 1994 the Office of Alternative Medicine (OAM)—now the National Center for Complementary and Alternative Medicine <http://www.nccam.nih.gov>—collaborated with the FDA <http://www.fda.gov/> to evaluate the safety and efficacy of acupuncture needles. The Workshop on Acupuncture was held April 21-22, 1994, with more than 100 participants, including FDA staff, official representatives of many national and international acupuncture organizations, and acupuncture researchers.

### National Institutes of Health Consensus Statement on Acupuncture

NIH consensus statements are prepared by a non-advocate, non-federal panel of experts, based on presentations by investigators working in areas relevant to the consensus. On November 5, 1997, the panel that convened to consider acupuncture produced the following statement:

"Acupuncture as a therapeutic intervention is widely practiced in the United States. While there have been many studies of its potential usefulness, many of these studies provide equivocal results because of design, sample size, and other factors. The issue is further complicated by inherent difficulties in the use of appropriate controls, such as placebos and sham acupuncture groups. However, promising results have emerged, for example, showing efficacy of acupuncture in adult post-operative and chemotherapy nausea and vomiting and in post-operative dental pain. There are other situations such as addiction, stroke rehabilitation, headache, menstrual cramps, tennis elbow, fibromyalgia, myofacial pain, osteoarthritis, low back pain, carpal tunnel syndrome, and asthma where acupuncture may be useful as an adjunct treatment or an acceptable alternative or be included in a comprehensive management program. Further research is likely to uncover additional areas where acupuncture interventions will be useful."

More information on the statement, including the full text, program and abstracts from the meeting, bibliography, and related publications and all materials ordering information, is available at <http://odp.od.nih.gov/consensus/cons/107/107_intro.htm> (Fig. 5-1).

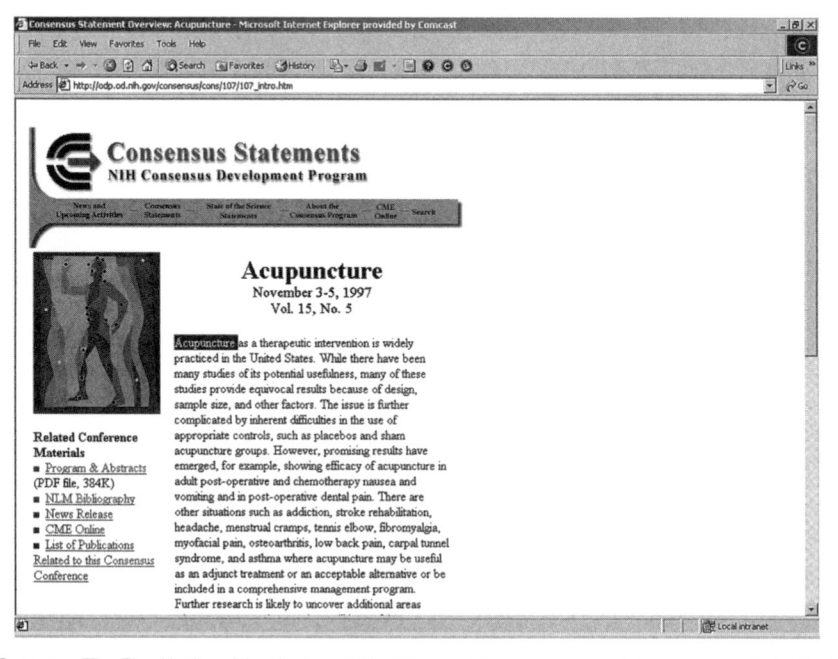

FIG. 5-1  ■  The National Institutes of Health provides consensus statements on its Web site.

## Abstracts of Cochrane Collaboration Systematic Reviews

Abstracts of systematic reviews of the literature on acupuncture are available from the Cochrane Collaboration at **<http://www.update-software.com/Cochrane/default.HTM>** (Fig. 5-2.).

## Evidence-Based Summaries from Bandolier

Table 5-1 lists evidence-based summaries from Bandolier describing the effects of acupuncture on various conditions (Fig. 5-3).

## British Medical Journal Collected Resources

ABC of Complementary Medicine: Acupuncture
Andrew Vickers and Catherine Zollman
*BMJ* 319:973-976, 1999
http://bmj.com/cgi/content/full/319/7215/973

## BioMed Central Articles

The following resources are available from the BioMed Central (BMC) Web site (Fig. 5-4):
**Electroacupuncture Versus Diclofenac in Symptomatic Treatment of Osteoarthritis of the Knee: a Randomized Controlled Trial**
Chaichan Sangdee and others

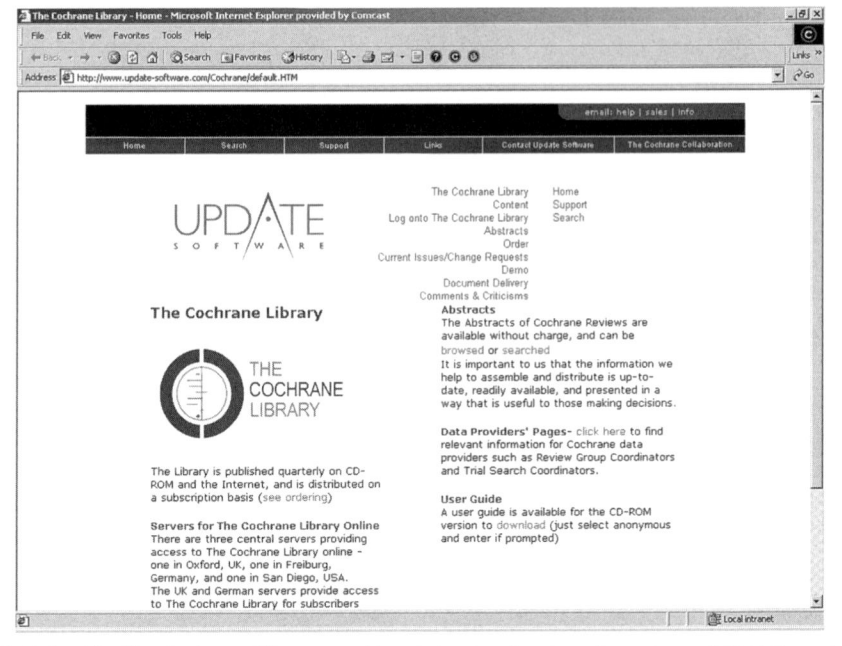

FIG. 5-2 ■ The Cochrane Library provides abstracts of systematic reviews of CAM therapies.

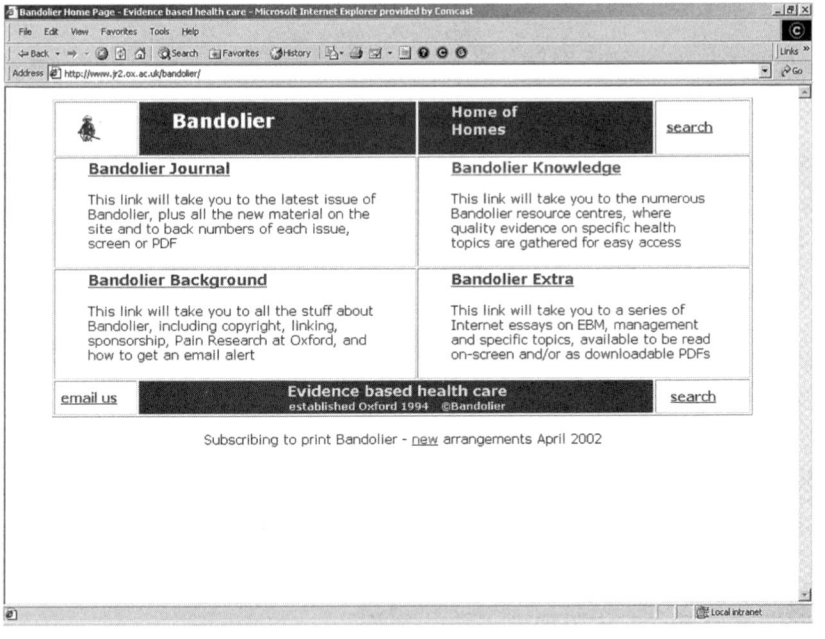

FIG. 5-3 ■ Bandolier provides evidence-based summaries of the effects of CAM on various conditions.

**TABLE 5-1** Evidence-Based Summaries from Bandolier on the Efficacy of Acupuncture

| CONDITION | URL | REFERENCE |
|---|---|---|
| Asthma | http://www.jr2.ox.ac.uk/ bandolier/booth/ alternat/AT002.html | Linde K, Jobst K, Panton J: Acupuncture for chronic asthma (Cochrane review). In the *Cochrane Library*, issue 1, Oxford, 2000, Update Software. |
| Back pain | http://www.jr2.ox.ac.uk/ bandolier/band60/ b60-2.html | Ernst E, White AR: Acupuncture for back pain: a meta-analysis of randomised controlled trials, *Arch Intern Med* 158:2235-2241, 1998. |
| Back and neck pain | http://www.jr2.ox.ac.uk/ bandolier/booth/ alternat/CP097.html | Ernst E, White AR: Acupuncture for back pain: a meta-analysis of randomised controlled trials, *Arch Intern Med* 158:2235-2241, 1998. White AR, Ernst E: A systematic review of randomised controlled trials of acupuncture for neck pain, *Rheumatology* 38:143-147, 1999. |
| Fibromyalgia | http://www.jr2.ox.ac.uk/ bandolier/band90/ b90-3.html | Berman BM and others: Is acupuncture effective in the treatment of fibromyalgia? *J Fam Pract* 48:213-218, 1999. Deluze C and others: Electroacupuncture in fibromyalgia: results of a controlled trial, *BMJ* 305:1249-1252, 1992. |
| Nausea and vomiting after surgery | http://www.jr2.ox.ac.uk/ bandolier/band71/ b71-9.html | Lee A, Done ML: The use of nonpharmacological techniques to prevent postoperative nausea and vomiting: a meta-analysis, *Anesth Analg* 88:1362-1369, 1999. |
| Osteoarthritis | http://www.jr2.ox.ac.uk/ bandolier/booth/ alternat/AT008.html | Ernst E: Acupuncture as a symptomatic treatment of osteoarthritis: a systematic review, *Scand J Rheumatol* 26:444-447, 1997. |
| Recurrent headache | http://www.jr2.ox.ac.uk/ bandolier/booth/ alternat/AT003.html | Melchart D and others: Acupuncture for recurrent headaches: a systematic review of randomized controlled trials, *Cephalalgia* 19(9):779-786, 1999. |
| Smoking cessation | http://www.jr2.ox.ac.uk/ bandolier/band72/ b72-5.html | White AR, Rampes H, Ernst E: Acupuncture for smoking cessation (Cochrane review). In *Cochrane Library*, issue 1, Oxford, 2000, Update Software. White AR, Resch KL, Ernst E: A meta-analysis of acupuncture techniques for smoking cessation, *Tob Control* 8:393-397, 1999. |
| Temporomandibular joint dysfunction | http://www.jr2.ox.ac.uk/ bandolier/booth/ alternat/AT005.html | Ernst E, White AR: Acupuncture as a treatment for temporomandibular joint dysfunction: a systematic review of randomised trials, *Arch Otolaryngol Head Neck Surg* 125:269-272, 1999. |

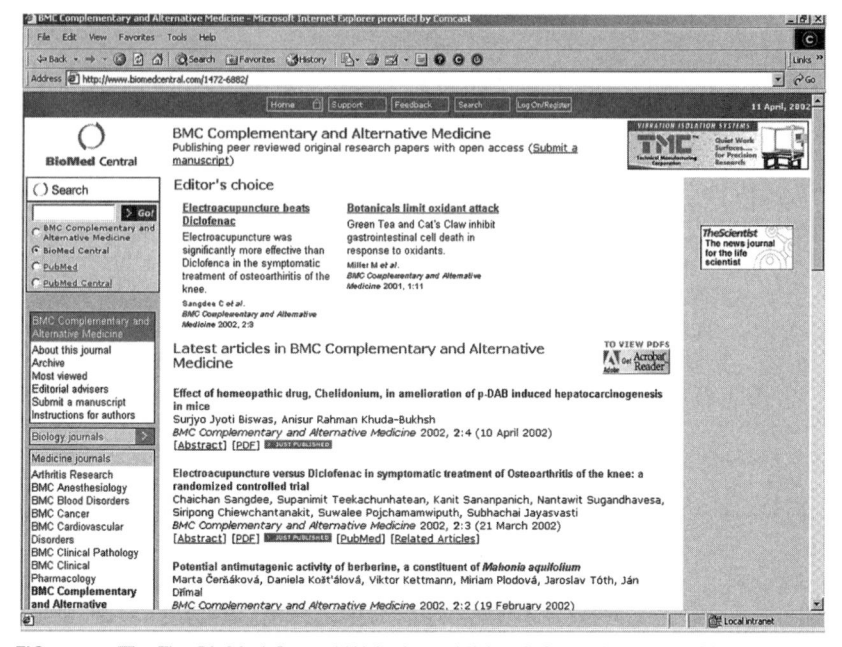

**FIG. 5-4** ■ The BioMed Central Web site publishes information about CAM therapies.

*BMC Complementary and Alternative Medicine* 2:3, 2002 (accessed March 21, 2002)
http://www.biomedcentral.com/1472-6882/
**Systematic Reviews of Complementary Therapies: An Annotated Bibliography. Part 1. Acupuncture**
Klaus Linde and others
*BMC Complementary and Alternative Medicine* 1:3, 2001 (accessed July 16, 2001)

## Books

*Acupuncture: A Comprehensive Text (Shanghai College of Traditional Chinese Medicine)*
John Bensky and Dan O'Connor
Eastlant Press, 1981
*Acupuncture Efficacy: A Compendium of Controlled Clinical Studies*
Stephen Birch and Richard Hammerschlag
National Academy of Acupuncture and Oriental Medicine, 1996
*Acupuncture Energetics: A Clinical Approach for Physicians*
Joseph M. Helms
Medical Acupuncture, 1996

*Acupuncture, Trigger Points, and Musculoskeletal Pain*
P.F. Baldry
Churchill Livingstone, 1993
**Basics of Acupuncture**
Gabriel Stux and Bruce Pomerantz
Springer Verlag, 1998
*Chinese Acupuncture and Moxibustion*
Cheng Xin-nong
China Books & Periodicals, April 2000
*Clinical Acupuncture*
Gabriel Stux, R. Hammershlag, and B.M. Berman
Churchill Livingstone, 2000
*Color Atlas of Acupuncture: Body Points, Ear Points, Trigger Points*
Hans-Ulrich Hecker and others
Thieme Medical Publishers, 2001
*Foundations of Chinese Medicine*
Giovanni Maciocia
Churchill Livingstone, 1997
*Medical Acupuncture*
J. Filshie and A. White
Churchill Livingstone, 1997
*Scientific Basis of Acupuncture*
Gabriel Stux and others, editors
Springer Verlag, 2000
*The Web That Has No Weaver*
Ted Kaptchuck
Contemporary Books, 2000

## Journals

*Acupuncture and Electro-Therapeutics*
http://www.geocities.com/icaet/seminars.html
*Acupuncture in Medicine*
http://www.medical-acupuncture.co.uk/aimintro.htm
*Chinese Journal of Integrated Traditional and Western Medicine*
http://www.relaxingnaturalhealth.com/
*International Journal of Clinical Acupuncture*
http://www.allertonpress.com/journals/acup.htm
*Journal of Chinese Medicine*
http://www.jcm.co.uk/
*Medical Acupuncture*
http://www.medicalacupuncture.org/
*NAAOM Journal*
http://www.naaom.org/journal.html

## Professional Organizations

American Academy of Medical Acupuncture (AAMA)
http://www.medicalacupuncture.org/
American Association of Oriental Medicine (AAOM)
http://www.aaom.org/
British Acupuncture Council
http://www.acupuncture.org.uk
British Medical Acupuncture Society
http://www.medical-acupuncture.co.uk
Foundation for Traditional Chinese Medicine
http://www.ftcm.org.uk/
Medical Acupuncture Research Foundation
http://www.medicalacupuncture.org/
National Acupuncture and Oriental Medicine Alliance
http://www.acuall.org/
Society for Acupuncture Research (SAR)
http://www.acupunctureresearch.org/

## ■ HERBAL MEDICINE

Herbal medicine is thriving in Europe and the United States. The sale of herbal medicines is one of the fastest growing industries in the United States, with more than $5 billion in sales annually. Herbal therapies are sold in pharmacies and health food stores, and herbal therapies on the Internet increasingly are used by matching selected herbal preparations with particular diseases or symptoms.

### Abstracts of Cochrane Collaboration Systematic Reviews

Abstracts of systematic reviews of the literature on herbal medicine are available from the Cochrane Collaboration at <**http://www.update-software.com/Cochrane/ default.HTM**>.

### Evidence-Based Summaries from Bandolier

Table 5-2 lists evidence-based summaries from Bandolier describing the effects of herbal medicines on various conditions.

### British Medical Journal Collected Resources

The Collected Resources of the *British Medical Journal* can be found at <**http://bmj.com**> (Fig. 5-5).
Adverse Reactions to Watch for in Patients Using Herbal Remedies
R. Ko
*West J Med* 171:181-186, 1999
http://www.ewjm.com/cgi/reprint/171/3/181

**TABLE 5-2** Evidence-Based Summaries from Bandolier on the Efficacy of Herbal Medicine and Phytomedicine

| SUMMARY TITLE | URL | REFERENCE |
|---|---|---|
| Aloe vera effectiveness for psoriasis and genital herpes | http://www.jr2.ox.ac.uk/ bandolier/booth/ alternat/AT125.html | Vogler BK, Ernst E: Aloe vera: a systematic review of its clinical effectiveness, *Br J Gen Pract* 49:823-828, 1999. |
| Artemether for severe malaria | http://www.jr2.ox.ac.uk/ bandolier/booth/ alternat/AT127.html | Pittler MH, Ernst E: Artemether for severe malaria: a meta-analysis of randomised clinical trials, *Chronic Infect Dis* 28:597-601, 1999. |
| Artichoke for cholesterol reduction | http://www.jr2.ox.ac.uk/ bandolier/booth/ alternat/AT033.html | Pittler MH, Ernst E: Artichoke leaf extract for serum cholesterol reduction, *Perfusion* 11:338-340. 1998. |
| β-Sitosterol for benign prostatic hyperplasia | http://www.jr2.ox.ac.uk/ bandolier/band92/ b92-4.html | Wilt TJ and others: β-Sitosterol for the treatment of benign prostatic hyperplasia: a systematic review, *BJU Int* 83:976-983, 1999. |
| Cernilton for benign prostatic hyperplasia | http://www.jr2.ox.ac.uk/ bandolier/booth/Mens/ Cern.html | MacDonal R and others: A systematic review of cernilton for the treatment of benign prostatic hyperplasia, *BJU Int* 85:836-841, 1999. |
| Chinese herbal medicine for irritable bowel disease | http://www.jr2.ox.ac.uk/ bandolier/band60/ b60-7.html | Bensoussan A and others: Treatment of irritable bowel syndrome with Chinese herbal medicine: a randomized controlled study, *JAMA* 280:1585-1589, 1998. |
| Chinese herbal medicine for eczema | http://www.jr2.ox.ac.uk/ bandolier/booth/ alternat/AT021.html | Armstrong NC, Ernst E: The treatment of eczema with Chinese herbs: a systematic review of randomized clinical trials, *Br J Clin Pharmacol* 48:262-264, 1999. |
| Chinese herbal medicine for respiratory tract infection | http://www.jr2.ox.ac.uk/ bandolier/booth/ alternat/AT131.html | Lui C, Douglas RM: Chinese herbal medicine in the treatment of acute respiratory tract infections: review of randomised controlled clinical trials, *Clin Infect Dis* 28:235-236, 1999. |
| Chinese herbs for hepatitis B | http://www.jr2.ox.ac.uk/ bandolier/booth/ alternat/cherbhepat.html | Lui JP, McIntosh H, Lin H: Chinese medicinal herbs for chronic hepatitis B (Cochrane Review). In the *Cochrane Library,* issue 1, 2001, Oxford, Update Software. |
| Cranberry juice and urinary tract infections | http://www.jr2.ox.ac.uk/ bandolier/band6/ b6-3.html | Avorn J and others: Reduction of bacteriuria and pyuria after ingestion of cranberry juice, *JAMA* 271:751, 1994. |
| Echinacea for the common cold | http://www.jr2.ox.ac.uk/ bandolier/booth/ alternat/echinaceacold. html | Barrett B, Vohmann M, Calabrese C: Echinacea for upper respiratory infection, *J Fam Pract* 48:628-635, 1999. |

*Continued*

 **TABLE 5-2** Evidence-Based Summaries from Bandolier on the Efficacy of Herbal Medicine and Phytomedicine—cont'd

| SUMMARY TITLE | URL | REFERENCE |
|---|---|---|
| Evening primrose oil for premenstrual syndrome | http://www.jr2.ox.ac.uk/bandolier/booth/alternat/AT058.html | Budeiri D, Li Wan Po A, Dornan JC: Is evening primrose oil of value in the treatment of premenstrual syndrome? *Control Clin Trials* 17:60-68, 1996. Melanby A, Best L, Stevens A: *Evening primrose oil for cyclical mastalgia.* Development and Evaluation Committee Report No. 65, December 1996. Research and Development Directorate, Wessex Institute for Health Research and Development. |
| Evening primrose oil and fish oil for schizophrenia | http://www.jr2.ox.ac.uk/bandolier/booth/alternat/evprimschiz.html | Joy CB, Mumby-Croft R, Joy LA: Poly-unsaturated fatty acid (fish or evening primrose oil) for schizophrenia (Cochrane review). In the *Cochrane Library,* issue 3, Oxford, 2000, Update Software. |
| Feverfew for preventing migraine | http://www.jr2.ox.ac.uk/bandolier/band65/b65-9.html | Vogler BK, Pittler MH, Ernst E: Feverfew as a preventive treatment for migraine: a systematic review, *Cephalalgia* 18:704-708, 1998. |
| Garlic for blood pressure | http://www.jr2.ox.ac.uk/bandolier/booth/alternat/AT025.html | Silagy C, Neil A: A meta-analysis of the effect of garlic on blood pressure, *J Hypertension* 12(4):463-468, 1994. |
| Garlic for hyperlipidemia | http://www.jr2.ox.ac.uk/bandolier/booth/alternat/AT054.html | Silagy C, Neil A: Garlic as a lipid lowering agent: a meta-analysis, *J R Coll Physicians Lond* 28(1):39-45, 1994. |
| Ginger for nausea and vomiting | http://www.jr2.ox.ac.uk/bandolier/booth/alternat/AT128.html | Ernst E, Pittler MH: Efficacy of ginger for nausea and vomiting: a systematic review of randomised clinical trials, *Br J Anaesth* 84(3):367-371, 2000. |
| Ginkgo for dementia | http://www.jr2.ox.ac.uk/bandolier/booth/alternat/AT123.html | Ernst E, Pittler MH: *Ginkgo biloba* for dementia: a systematic review of double-blind, placebo-controlled trials, *Clin Drug Invest* 17:301-308, 1999. |
| Ginkgo for tinnitus | http://www.jr2.ox.ac.uk/bandolier/booth/alternat/AT124.html | Ernst E, Stevinson C: *Ginkgo biloba* for tinnitus: a review, *Clin Otolaryngol* 24:164-167, 1999. |
| Ginseng for vitality | http://www.jr2.ox.ac.uk/bandolier/band71/b71-5.html | Volger BK, Pittler MH, Ernst E: The efficacy of ginseng: a systematic review of randomised clinical trials, *Eur J Clin Pharmacol* 55:567-575, 1999. |
| Green tea and risk of gastric cancer | http://www.jr2.ox.ac.uk/bandolier/booth/hliving/greentea.html | Tsubono Y and others: Green tea and the risk of gastric cancer in Japan, *N Engl J Med* 344:632-636, 2001. |

## TABLE 5-2 Evidence-Based Summaries from Bandolier on the Efficacy of Herbal Medicine and Phytomedicine—cont'd

| SUMMARY TITLE | URL | REFERENCE |
|---|---|---|
| Horse chestnut relieves chronic venous insufficiency | http://www.jr2.ox.ac.uk/bandolier/booth/alternat/AT132.html | Pittler MH, Ernst E: Horse-chestnut for chronic venous insufficiency: a criteria-based systematic review, *Arch Dermatol* 134:1356-1360, 1998. |
| Kava extract reduces anxiety | http://www.jr2.ox.ac.uk/bandolier/booth/alternat/AT126.html | Pittler MH, Ernst E: Efficacy of kava extract for treating anxiety: systematic review and meta-analysis, *J Clin Psychopharmacol* 20(1):84-89, 2000. |
| Peppermint oil for irritable bowel syndrome | http://www.jr2.ox.ac.uk/bandolier/booth/alternat/AT022.html | Pittler MH, Ernst E: Peppermint oil for irritable bowel syndrome: a critical review and meta-analysis, *Am J Gastroenterol* 93(7):1131-1135, 1998. |
| Phytodolor for musculoskeletal pain | http://www.jr2.ox.ac.uk/bandolier/booth/alternat/AT026.html | Ernst E: The efficacy of Phytodolor for the treatment of musculoskeletal pain: a systematic review of randomized clinical trials, *Nat Med J* 2(5):14-17, 1999. |
| *Pygeum africanum* for benign prostatic hyperplasia | http://www.jr2.ox.ac.uk/bandolier/booth/Mens/Pyaf.html | Ishani A and others: *Pygeum africanum* for the treatment of patients with benign prostatic hyperplasia: a systematic review and quantitative meta-analysis, *Am J Med* 109:654-664, 2000. |
| St John's wort for depression | http://www.jr2.ox.ac.uk/bandolier/band31/b31-2.html | Linde K and others: St John's wort for depression: an overview and meta-analysis of randomised clinical trials, *BMJ* 313:253-258, 1996. |
| Saw palmetto and prostatic hypertrophy | http://www.jr2.ox.ac.uk/bandolier/band73/b73-2.html | Wilt TJ and others: Saw palmetto extracts for treatment of benign prostatic hyperplasia: a systematic review, *JAMA* 280:1604-1609, 1998. Wilt T and others: *Serenoa repens* for benign prostatic hyperplasia (Cochrane review). In the *Cochrane Library*, issue 1, Oxford, 2000, Update Software. |
| Soya is helpful in menopause | http://www.jr2.ox.ac.uk/bandolier/band56/b56-3.html | Seidl MM, Stewart DE: Alternative treatments for menopausal symptoms: systematic review of scientific and lay literature, *Can Fam Physician* 44:1299-1308, 1998. |
| Valerian for insomnia | http://www.jr2.ox.ac.uk/bandolier/band81/b81-7.html | Stevinson C, Ernst E: Valerian for insomnia: a systematic review of randomized clinical trials, *Sleep Med* 1:91-99, 2000. |
| Yohimbine for erectile dysfunction | http://www.jr2.ox.ac.uk/bandolier/booth/alternat/AT031.html | Ernst E, Pittler MH: Yohimbine for erectile dysfunction: a systematic review and meta-analysis of randomized clinical trials, *J Urol* 159:433-436, 1998. |

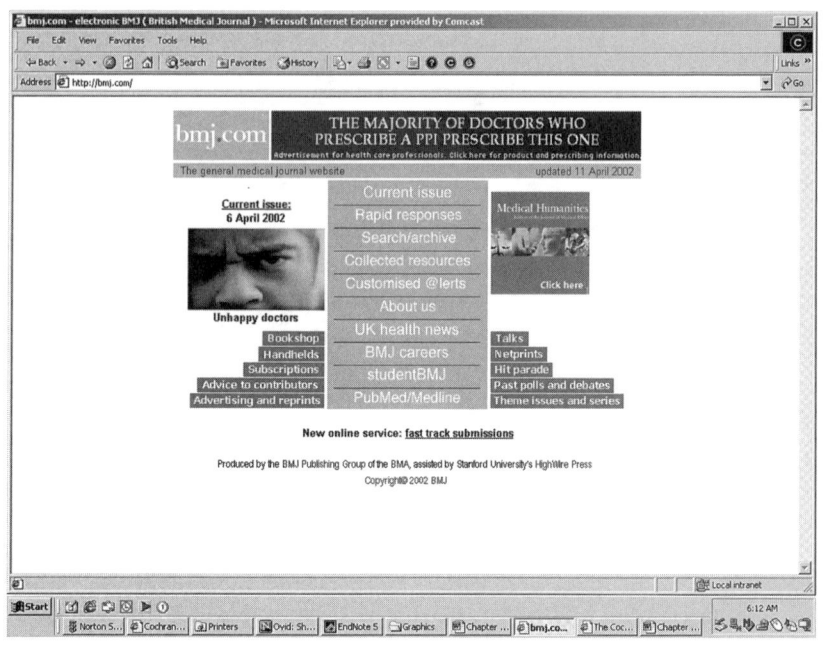

**FIG. 5-5**  ■  The Web site of the *British Medical Journal* offers a number of resources on CAM therapies.

## An Evidence-Based Review of the 10 Most Commonly Used Herbs
C. Mar and S. Bent
*West J Med* 171:168-171, 1999
http://www.ewjm.com/cgi/reprint/171/3/168.pdf
### Herbal Medicine
Andrew Vickers, Catherine Zollman, and Roberta Lee
*West J Med* 175:125-128, 2001
http://www.ewjm.com/cgi/content/full/175/2/125
### Herbal Medicine: A Practical Guide to Safety and Quality Assurance
M.D. Rotblatt
*West J Med* 171:172-175, 1999
http:www.ewjm/com/cgi/reprint/171/3/172
### Herbal Medicines for Asthma: A Systematic Review
A. Huntley and E. Ernst
*Thorax* 55:925-929, 2000
http://thorax.bmjjournals.com/cgi/content/full/55/11/925

### Books

*British Herbal Pharmacopoeia*
British Herbal Medicine Association, 1996
Monographs cover identification and standards for plant materials used in herbal
products.

*The Complete German Commission E Monographs: Therapeutic Guide to Herbal Medicines*
Mark Blumenthal
American Botanical Council, 1998
This collection, translated from the original German monographs, contains authoritative information on the safety and efficacy of herbs and phytomedicinals as well as a wealth of extra data.

*Encyclopedia of Common Natural Ingredients Used in Food, Drugs, and Cosmetics*
Wiley, 1995
This encyclopedia is an invaluable research resource for those involved in the manufacture and research of natural products.

*ESCOP Monographs*
A.Y. Leung and S. Foster
European Scientific Cooperative on Phytotherapy, from 1996 to the present
This work contains six fascicles on the medicinal uses of plant drugs, covering the top 50 herbs and phytomedicines in Europe, and is prepared by herbal experts from European academia and industry.

*Herb Contraindications and Drug Interactions,* ed. 2
Mark Blumenthal
Eclectic Medical Publications, 1998
Warnings and interactions are documented for 181 herbs, and appendixes are included.

*Herbal Medicine: Expanded Commission E Monographs*
Francis Brinker
Integrative Medicine Communications, 1999
This new and updated reference is based on the original translation from German by Mark Blumenthal.

*PDR for Herbal Medicines,* ed. 2
Medical Economics Company, 2000
This text offers authoritative information from the company that produces the *Physician's Desk Reference.*

*WHO Monographs on Selected Medicinal Plants*
World Health Organization, 1999
This collection of 28 monographs covers quality control and traditional and clinical uses of medicinal plants, particularly in countries that rely heavily on these plants for primary health care.

## Journals

*The European Phytojournal*
http://info.ex.ac.uk/phytonet/phytojournal
*Fitoterapia*
http://www.elsevier.com/locate/issn/0367326x
*HerbalGram*
http://www.herbalgram.org/
*Journal of Ethnopharmacology*
http://www.elsevier.nl/inca/publications/store/5/0/6/0/3/5/

*Journal of Naturopathic Medicine*
http://www.healthy.net/library/journals/naturopathic/index.html
*Phytochemistry*
http://www.elsevier.nl/inca/publications/store/2/7/3/

## Professional Organizations

**American Botanical Council (ABC)**
http://www.herbalgram.org/
**American Herbalists Guild**
http://www.healthy.net/herbalists/
**Herb Research Foundation**
http://www.herbs.org/index.html
**Herb Society home page (United Kingdom)**
http://www.herbsociety.co.uk/
**Herb Society of America**
http://www.herbsociety.org/

## Internet Resources

**Botanical.com**
http://www.botanical.com/
**Botanical Enterprises, Inc.**
http://www.bei-botanicals.com/
**CyberBotanica**
http://biotech.icmb.utexas.edu/
**GRIN Taxonomy**
http://www.ars-grin.gov/npgs/tax/taxgenform.html
**HerbMed**
http://www.herbmed.org/
**Longwood Herbal Task Force**
http://www.mcp.edu/herbal/
**Medherb.com**
http://medherb.com/
**MedWebPlus—Herbs**
MedWebPlus offers a categorized collection of herbal sites
http://www.medwebplus.com/subject/Medicine,_Herbal.html
**Michael Tierra's Planetary Herbology**
http://www.planetherbs.com/
**Phytochemical and Ethnobotanical Databases**
http://www.ars-grin.gov/duke/
**Phytotherapies.org**
http://www.phytotherapies.org/
**Rocky Mountain Herbal Institute**
http://www.rmhiherbal.org/

MANUAL THERAPIES

Manual therapies such as chiropractic, osteopathy, and massage are based on manipulation or movement of the body. For example, chiropractic and osteopathy are considered manipulative therapies and focus on the relationship between structure (primarily the spine) and function and how that relationship affects the preservation and restoration of health. In the United States the practice of osteopathy has embraced the modern allopathic medical model, so we will focus on chiropractic and massage. Massage therapists manipulate the soft tissues of the body to normalize those tissues. In doing so, massage therapists seek to promote health and treat illness through the alleviation of physical tension in the body.

## Chiropractic Guidelines

An exhaustive review of chiropractic by the Agency for Health Care Policy and Research (AHCPR) and published by the National Technical Information Service (NTIS) includes information on all aspects of chiropractic, including history, belief systems, content of practice, research, benefits, and possible risks associated with spinal manipulation. (The full-text version is available at <**http://www.chiroweb. com/archives/ahcpr/uschiros.htm**>.)

## Abstracts of Cochrane Collaboration Systematic Reviews

Abstracts of systematic reviews of the literature on manual therapies are available from the Cochrane Collaboration at <**http://www.update-software.com/Cochrane/ default.HTM**>.

## Evidence–Based Summaries from Bandolier

Table 5-3 lists evidence-based summaries from Bandolier describing the effects of manual therapies on various conditions.

## British Medical Journal Collected Resources

**ABC of Complementary Medicine: Massage Therapies**
Andrew Vickers and Catherine Zollman
*BMJ* 319:1254-1257, 1999.
**ABC of Complementary Medicine: The Manipulative Therapies—Osteopathy and Chiropractic**
Andrew Vickers and Catherine Zollman
*BMJ* 319:1176-1179, 1999
http://bmj.com/cgi/content/full/319/7218/1176
**ACC Position Paper: Issues in Chiropractic**
The position paper is from the Association of Chiropractic Colleges on the profession of chiropractic.
http://www.chirocolleges.org/paradigm_scopet.html

 **TABLE 5-3** Evidence-Based Summaries from Bandolier on the Efficacy of Manual Therapies

| TYPE OF THERAPY | URL | REFERENCE |
|---|---|---|
| Cervical spine manipulation and mobilization for neck pain and headache | http://www.jr2.ox.ac.uk/bandolier/booth/alternat/CP095.html | Hurwitz EL and others: Manipulation and mobilization of the cervical spine: a systematic review of the literature, *Spine* 21(15):1746-1760, 1996. |
| Massage for growth and development of preterm infants | http://www.jr2.ox.ac.uk/bandolier/booth/alternat/Massaginfant.html | Vickers A and others: Massage for promoting growth and development in low birth-weight infants (Cochrane review). In the *Cochrane Library*, issue 1, Oxford, 2001, Update Software. |
| Abdominal massage for chronic constipation | http://www.jr2.ox.ac.uk/bandolier/booth/alternat/AT043.html | Ernst E: Abdominal massage for chronic constipation: a systematic review of controlled clinical trials, *Forsch Komplementarmed* 6:149-151, 1999. |
| Effectiveness of massage | http://www.jr2.ox.ac.uk/bandolier/booth/alternat/AT045.html | Ernst E: Clinical effectiveness of massage: a critical review, *Forsch Komplementarmed* 1:226-232, 1994. |
| Effleurage backrub for relaxation | http://www.jr2.ox.ac.uk/bandolier/booth/alternat/AT046.html | Labyak SE, Metzger BL: The effects of effleurage backrub on the physiological components of relaxation: a meta-analysis, *Nurs Res* 46:59-62, 1997. |
| Massage for lower back pain | http://www.jr2.ox.ac.uk/bandolier/booth/alternat/AT042.html | Ernst E: Massage therapy for low back pain: a systematic review, *J Pain Symptom Manage* 17:56-69, 1999. |
| Massage for delayed-onset muscle soreness | http://www.jr2.ox.ac.uk/bandolier/booth/alternat/AT044.html | Ernst E: Does post-exercise massage treatment reduce delayed onset muscle soreness? *Br J Sports Med* 32:212-214, 1998. |

## Books on Chiropractic

*Basic Chiropractic Procedural Manual*
R.C. Schafer
American Chiropractic Association Foundation, 1984
*Chiropractic Approach to Head Pain*
Darryl D. Curl
Lippincott Williams & Wilkins, 1994
*Differential Diagnosis for the Chiropractor: Protocols and Algorithms*
Thomas A. Souza
Aspen, 1998

*Tendon and Ligament Healing: A New Approach Through Manual Therapy*
William Weintraub
American Chiropractic Association Foundation, 1986

## Books on Massage Therapy

*Massage Therapy Career Guide: For Hands-on Success*
Steve Capelli
Delmar Publishers, 1998
*Massage Therapy: Principles and Practice*
Susan Salvo and Maureen Pfeiffer
Harcourt, 1999
*Milady's Theory and Practice of Therapeutic Massage*
Mark Beck
Delmar Publishers, 1999
*Mosby's Fundamentals of Therapeutic Massage*
Sandy Fritz
Harcourt, 1999

## Chiropractic Journals

*Journal of the American Chiropractic Association*
http://www.amerchiro.org/publications/
*Journal of Bodywork and Movement Therapies*
http://www.harcourt-international.com/journals/jbmt
*Journal of Manipulative and Physiological Therapeutics*
http://www.2.us.elsevierhealth.com/scripts/om.dll/serve?action=sea
*Massage Therapy Journal*
http://www.amtamassage.org/journal

## Professional and Referral Organizations

American Chiropractic Association (ACA)
http://www.amerchiro.org/
American Massage Therapy Association (AMTA)
http://www.amtamassage.org/
American Oriental Bodywork Therapy Association (AOBTA)
http://www.healthy.net/aobta
Association of Chiropractic Colleges
http://www.chirocolleges.org/
International Chiropractic Association
http://www.chiropractic.org/
National Certification Board for Therapeutic Massage and Bodywork (NCBTMB)
http://www.ncbtmb.com/

## Internet Resources

### Chiropractic

Chiropractic Online Today
http://www.chiro-online.com/
ChiroWeb
http://www.chiroweb.com/

### Massage

American Massage Therapy Association
http://www.amtamassage.org/
Feldenkrais Resources
http://www.feldenkrais-resources.com/
American Society for the Alexander Technique
http://www.alexandertech.com/
MassageTherapy.com
http://www.massagetherapy.com/
Massage Therapy home page
http://www.lightlink.com/massage/index.html
Massage Therapy Web Central
http://www.qwl.com/mts.html
Rolf Institute of Structural Integration
http://www.rolf.org/index.html
University of Michigan "Muscles in Action"
http://www.med.umich.edu/lrc/Hypermuscle/Hyper.html

## References

1. The Landmark Report II on HMOs and Alternative Therapy: 1999 nationwide HMO study of alternative care, *Landmark Healthcare*, 1999, *http://www.landmarkhealthcare.com*.
2. Goldbeck-Wood SDA and others: Complementary medicine is booming worldwide, *BMJ* 313(7050):131-133, 1996.
3. Vickers A: Recent advances: complementary medicine, *BMJ* 321(7262):683-686, 2000.

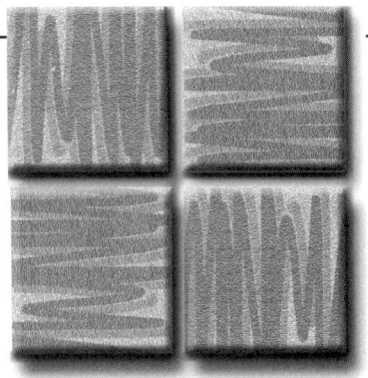

CHAPTER

# Complementary Therapies of the Body, Mind, and Spirit

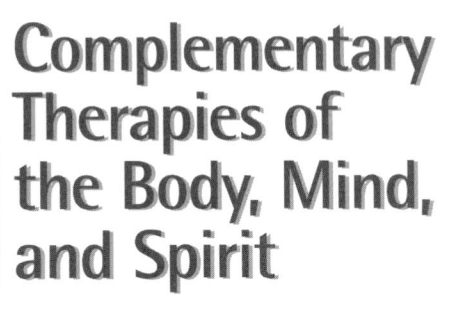

**Chapter Highlights**
Diet and Nutritional Therapies
Mind-Body Therapies
Homeopathy
Prayer, Spirituality, and Energetic Therapies

## ■ DIET AND NUTRITIONAL THERAPIES

Complementary nutritional therapies range from well-researched biochemical interventions that are prescribed by medical professionals, such as vitamin C and vitamin $B_6$, to unproven and potentially dangerous therapies and diets. In practice these interventions involve dietary supplementation or dietary modification in an effort to improve health or treat specific diseases. Some overlap exists between the herbal and nutritional interventions described in Chapter 5 and this chapter. In these areas of overlap the authors have included the overlapping items.

### Abstracts of Cochrane Collaboration Systematic Reviews

Abstracts of systematic reviews of the literature on diet and nutritional therapies are available from the Cochrane Collaboration at **<http://www.update-software.com/ Cochrane/default.HTM>**.

### Evidence-Based Summaries from Bandolier

Table 6-1 lists evidence-based summaries from Bandolier describing the effects of diet and nutritional therapies on various conditions.

### British Medical Journal Collected Resources

**ABC of Complementary Medicine: Unconventional Approaches to Nutritional Medicine**
Andrew Vickers and Catherine Zollman
*BMJ* 319:1419-1422, 1999.
http://bmj.com/cgi/content/full/319/7211/693

**TABLE 6-1** Evidence-Based Summaries from Bandolier on the Efficacy of Diet and Nutritional Therapies

| TYPE OF THERAPY | URL | REFERENCE |
|---|---|---|
| Alternatives for menopause | http://www.jr2.ox.ac.uk/ bandolier/band56/ b56-3.html | Seidl MM, Stewart DE: Alternative treatments for menopausal symptoms: systematic review of scientific and lay literature, *Can Fam Physician* 44:1299-1308, 1998. |
| Chitosan for weight loss | http://www.jr2.ox.ac.uk/ bandolier/booth/ alternat/AT027.html | Ernst E, Pittler MH: Chitosan as a treatment for body weight reduction? A meta-analysis, *Perfusion* 11:461-465, 1998. |
| Chondroitin sulfate for osteoarthritis | http://www.jr2.ox.ac.uk/ bandolier/booth/ Arthritis/CSOA.html | Leeb BF and others: A meta-analysis of chondroitin sulfate in the treatment of osteoarthritis, *J Rheumatol* 27:205-211, 2000. |
| Cranberry juice reduces bacteri-uria and pyuria | http://www.jr2.ox.ac.uk/ bandolier/band6/ b6-3.html | McMurdo MET and others: A cost-effectiveness study of the management of intractable urinary incontinence by urinary catheterisation or incontinence pads, *J Epidemiol Community Health* 46:222-226, 1992. Avorn J and others: Reduction of bacteriuria and pyuria after ingestion of cranberry juice, *JAMA* 271:751-754, 1994. |
| Evening primrose oil for premenstrual syndrome | http://www.jr2.ox.ac.uk/ bandolier/booth/ alternat/AT058.html | Budeiri D, Li Wan Po A, Dornan JC: Is evening primrose oil of value in the treatment of premenstrual syndrome? *Control Clin Trials* 17:60-68, 1996. Melanby A, Best L, Stevens A: *Evening primrose oil for cyclical mastalgia,* Development and Evaluation Committee Report No. 65, December 1996, Research and Development Directorate, Wessex Institute for Health Research and Development. |
| Garlic for blood pressure | http://www.jr2.ox.ac.uk/ bandolier/booth/ alternat/AT025.html | Silagy C, Neil A: A meta-analysis of the effect of garlic on blood pressure, *J Hypertension* 12(4):463-468, 1994. |
| Garlic for hyperlipidemia | http://www.jr2.ox.ac.uk/ bandolier/booth/ alternat/AT054.html | Silagy C, Neil A: Garlic as a lipid lowering agent: a meta-analysis, *J R Coll Physicians Lond* 28(1):39-45, 1994. |
| Glucosamine and arthritis | http://www.jr2.ox.ac.uk/ bandolier/band46/ b46-2.html | Towheed TE and others: Glucosamine therapy for treating osteoarthritis (Cochrane review). In the *Cochrane Library,* issue 1, Oxford, 2001, Update Software. McAlindon TE and others: Glucosamine and chondroitin for treatment of osteoarthritis: a systematic quality assessment and meta-analysis, *JAMA* 283:1469-1473, 2000. Reginster JY and others: Long-term effects of glucosamine sulphate on osteoarthritis progression: a randomised, placebo-controlled clinical trial, *Lancet* 357:251-256, 2001. |

| TABLE 6-1 Evidence-Based Summaries from Bandolier on the Efficacy of Diet and Nutritional Therapies—cont'd | | |
|---|---|---|
| TYPE OF THERAPY | URL | REFERENCE |
| Melatonin for jet lag | http://www.jr2.ox.ac.uk/ bandolier/band82/ b82-4.html | Spitzer RL and others: Jet lag: clinical features, validation of a new syndrome-specific scale, and a lack of response to melatonin in a randomized, double-blind trial, *Am J Psychiatr* 156:1392-1396, 1999. |
| Peppermint oil for irritable bowel syndrome | http://www.jr2.ox.ac.uk/ bandolier/booth/ alternat/AT022.html | Pittler MH, Ernst E: Peppermint oil for irritable bowel syndrome: a critical review and meta-analysis, *Am J Gastroenterol* 93(7):1131-1135, 1998. |
| Vitamin $B_6$ for premenstrual syndrome | http://www.jr2.ox.ac.uk/ bandolier/booth/ alternat/AT023.html | Wyatt KM and others: Efficacy of vitamin B-6 in the treatment of premenstrual syndrome: systematic review, *BMJ* 318:1375-1381, 1999. |
| Vitamin E improves tardive dyskinesia | http://www.jr2.ox.ac.uk/ bandolier/booth/ alternat/AT051.html | Soares KVS, McGrath JJ: Vitamin E for neuroleptic-induced tardive dyskinesia (Cochrane review). In the *Cochrane Library*, issue 3, Oxford, 2000, Update Software. |

**MEDLINEplus Health Information, National Library of Medicine** (Fig. 6-1)
Vitamin and mineral supplements
http://www.nlm.nih.gov/medlineplus/vitaminandmineralsupplements.html
**National Academy of Sciences, Institute of Medicine, Food and Nutrition Board**
http://www4.nas.edu/IOM/IOMHome.nsf/Pages/Food+and+Nutrition+Board

## Position Papers from the American Dietetic Association

**Nutrition fact sheets**
http://www.eatright.org/nfs/#Vitamins,_Minerals,_and_Functional_Foods
**Vitamin and mineral supplementation**
http://www.eatright.org/gifs/phytochemicals.pdf

## Books

*Foundations of Nutritional Medicine: A Sourcebook of Clinical Research*
Melvin R. Werbach
Third Line Press, 1997
*Nutraceuticals: The Complete Guide Encyclopedia of Supplements, Herbs, Vitamins, and Healing Foods*
Arthur Roberts
Penguin, 2001
*PDR for Nutritional Supplements*
Sheldon S. Hendler
Medical Economics, 2001

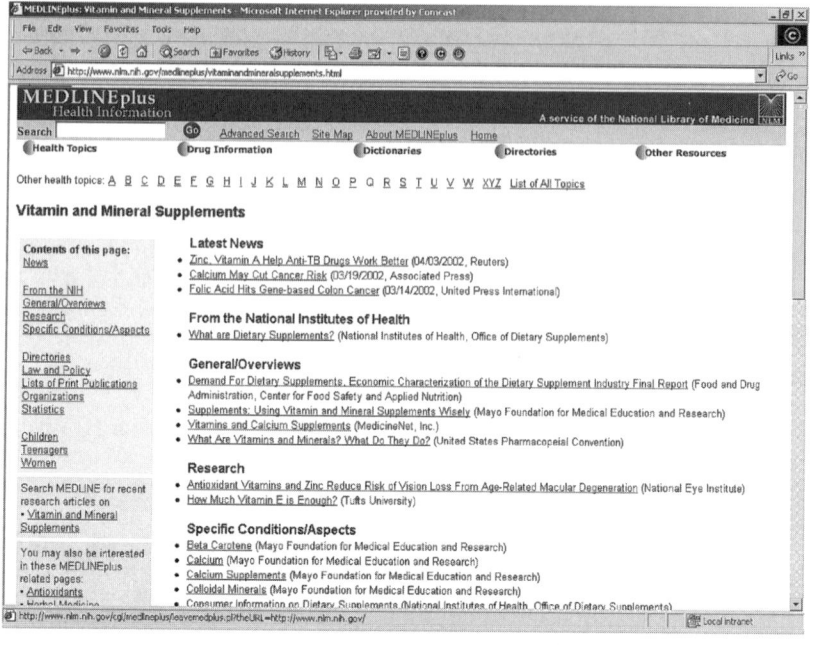

FIG. 6-1    ■    The MEDLINEplus Web site offers information on vitamin and mineral supplements.

*Vitamins, Herbs, Minerals, & Supplements: The Complete Guide*
H. Griffith Winter
Fisher Books, 1998
*Vitamins, Minerals, and Dietary Supplements*
American Dietetic Association and Marsha Hudnall
John Wiley & Sons, 1999

## Professional Organizations

**American Dietetic Association**
http://www.eatright.org
**American Nutraceutical Association**
http://www.americanutra.com/association.html

## Internet Resources

**Center for Science in the Public Interest**
http://www.cspinet.org/
**ConsumerLab.com**
http://www.consumerlab.com/
**Dietfraud.com**
http://www.dietfraud.com/
**Food and Nutrition Information Center (FNIC)**
http://www.nal.usda.gov/fnic/

**Healthwell**
http://www.healthwell.com/index.cfm
**International Bibliographic Information on Dietary Supplements Database**
http://ods.od.nih.gov/databases/ibids.html
**Macrobiotics On-Line**
http://www.kushiinstitute.org/
**MEDLINEplus**
http://www.nlm.nih.gov/medlineplus/foodnutritionandmetabolism.html
**The Natural Pharmacist**
http://tnp/com/
**Tufts University Nutrition Navigator**
http://navigator.tufts.edu/about.html
**United States Pharmacopeia (USP): Dietary Supplement Program**
http://www.usp.org/dietary/index.htm

## 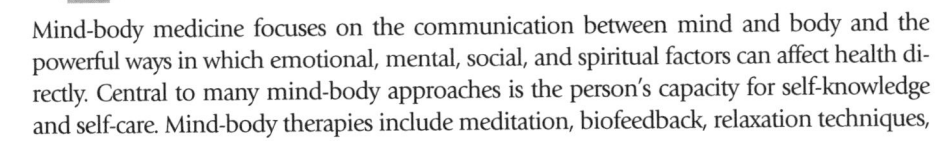 MIND–BODY THERAPIES

Mind-body medicine focuses on the communication between mind and body and the powerful ways in which emotional, mental, social, and spiritual factors can affect health directly. Central to many mind-body approaches is the person's capacity for self-knowledge and self-care. Mind-body therapies include meditation, biofeedback, relaxation techniques, music therapy, hypnosis, *qi gong,* and cognitive and behavioral interventions.

### Abstracts of Cochrane Collaboration Systematic Reviews

Abstracts of systematic reviews of the literature on diet and nutritional therapies are available from the Cochrane Collaboration at **<http://www.update-software.com/ Cochrane/default.HTM>**.

### Evidence–Based Summaries from Bandolier

Table 6-2 lists evidence-based summaries from Bandolier describing the effects of mind-body therapies on various conditions.

### British Medical Journal Collected Resources

**Hypnosis and Relaxation Therapies**
Andrew Vickers, Catherine Zollman, and David K. Payne
*West J Med* 175:269-272, 2001
http://www.ewjm.com/cgi/content/full/175/4/269

### Books

*The Healer Within: The New Medicine of Mind and Body*
Steven Locke
Plumsock Mesoamerican Studies, 1997
*Love, Medicine, and Miracles*
Bernie Siegal
Harper Perennial, 1990

**TABLE 6-2** Evidence-Based Summaries from Bandolier on the Efficacy of Mind-Body Interventions

| TYPE OF THERAPY | URL | REFERENCE |
|---|---|---|
| Biofeedback for anismus | http://www.jr2.ox.ac.uk/ bandolier/booth/ alternat/AT053.html | Ernst E, Resch KL: A meta-analysis of biofeedback treatment for anismus, *Eur J Phys Med* 5(5):157-159, 1995. |
| Breathing exercises for asthma | http://www.jr2.ox.ac.uk/ bandolier/booth/ alternat/ breathexasthma.html | Holloway E, Ram FSF: Breathing exercises for asthma (Cochrane review). In the *Cochrane Library,* issue 1, Oxford, 2001, Update Software. |
| Cognitive behavior therapy for chronic fatigue | http://www.jr2.ox.ac.uk/ bandolier/booth/ alternat/cbtfatigue. html | Price JR, Couper J: Cognitive behaviour therapy for adults with chronic fatigue syndrome (Cochrane review). In the *Cochrane Library,* issue 1, Oxford, 2001, Update Software. |
| Relaxation and music therapy for postoperative pain | http://www.jr2.ox.ac.uk/ bandolier/booth/ alternat/AT041.html | Good M: Effects of relaxation and music on postoperative pain: a review, *J Adv Nurs* 24:903-914, 1996. |
| Relaxation techniques | http://www.jr2.ox.ac.uk/ bandolier/band53/ b53-5.html | Seers K, Carroll D: Relaxation techniques for acute pain management: a systematic review, *J Adv Nurs* 27:466-475, 1998. Carroll D, Seers K: Relaxation techniques for chronic pain: a systematic review, *J Adv Nurs* 27:476-487, 1998. Moore RA and others: Quantitative systematic review of topically applied non-steroidal anti-inflammatory drugs, *BMJ* 316:333-338, 1998. |

*Mind as Healer, Mind as Slayer*
Ken Pelletier
Delta Books, 1984
*Mind-Body Medicine: A Clinician's Guide to Psychoneuroimmunology*
Allen Watkins
Harcourt Health Sciences Group, 1997
*Molecules of Emotion: Why You Feel the Way You Feel*
Candace B. Pert
Schribner, 1997
*Psychoneuroimmunology: An Interdisciplinary Introduction*
Manfred Schedlowski and Uwe Tewes
Academic Publishers, 1999
*Psychoneuroimmunology: The New Mind/Body Healing Program*
Elliot S. Dacher
Paragon House, 1991

## Journals

*Advances in Mind-Body Medicine*
http://www.harcourt-international.com/journals/
*Subtle Energies and Energy Medicine Journal*
http://www.issseem.org/journal.html

## Professional and Referral Organizations

**Academy for Guided Imagery**
http://www.healthy.net/agi
**American Association of Professional Hypnotherapists**
http://www.aaph.org
**American Psychotherapy and Medical Hypnosis Association**
http://apmha.com/
**Association for Applied Psychophysiology and Biofeedback**
http://www.aapb.org
**Center for Mind-Body Medicine**
http://www.cmbm.org/
**Center for Mindfulness in Medicine, Health Care, and Society**
University of Massachusetts Medical Center
http://www.umassmed.edu/cfm/
**International Association of Interactive Imagery**
http://www.iaii.org
**Mind-Body Medical Institute**
http://www.mbmi.org
**Transcendental Meditation Program**
http://www.tm.org

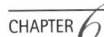 ## HOMEOPATHY

Homeopathy is a system of medicine that is based on the law of similars. The originator of homeopathy, Samuel Hahnemann, described this principle by using the Latin phrase *similia similibus curentur,* which translates "Let likes cure likes." Hahnemann further developed the principle into a system of healing. Homeopaths describe homeopathy as a system that attempts to stimulate the body to heal itself by using minute doses of plants, minerals, or other natural substances that are tailored to individuals and their illnesses.[1]

### Evidence-Based Summaries from Bandolier

Table 6-3 lists evidence-based summaries from Bandolier describing the effects of homeopathy on various conditions.

### British Medical Journal Collected Resources

ABC of Complementary Medicine: Homeopathy
Andrew Vickers and Catherine Zollman

*BMJ* 319:1115-1118, 1999.
http://bmj.com/cgi/content/full/319/7217/1115

## BioMed Central Article

A Systematic Review of the Quality of Homeopathic Clinical Trials
Wayne B. Jonas and others
*BMC Complementary and Alternative Medicine* 1:12, 2001
http://www.biomedcentral.com/1472-6882/1/12/

## Books

*Complete Guide to Homeopathy: The Principles and Practice of Treatment*
Andrew Lockie and Nicola Geddes
DK Publishing, 2000
*The Consumer's Guide to Homeopathy*
Dana Ullman
New York: Tarcher/Putnam, 1995
This is a user-friendly book to homeopathy with a solid review on homeopathic research.
*Cultured Mammalian Cells in Homeopathy Research: The Similia Principle in Self-Recovery*
Roeland van Wijk and Fred A.C. Wiegant
Utrecht: University of Utrecht, 1994
*Fundamental Research on Ultra-High Dilutions and Homeopathy*
P.C. Endler and J. Schulte (editors)
Dordrecht: Kluwer Academic, 1998
*Healing with Homeopathy*
Wayne B. Jonas, MD, and Jennifer Jacobs, MD
New York: Warner, 1996
*Homeopathy: A Frontier in Medical Science*
Paolo Bellavite and Andrea Signorini
Berkeley: North Atlantic, 1995
*Science of Homeopathy*
George Vithoulkas and William Tiller
Grove Press, 1980
*Ultra-High Dilution: Physiology and Physics*
Dordrecht: Kluwer Academic, 1994
A compilation of articles on basic science research. Very technical.
*Ultra-Low Doses*
M. Doutremepuich (editor)
Washington, DC/London: Taylor and Francis, 1991

## Journals

*British Homeopathic Journal*
http://www.elsevier-international.com/journals/homp/
*The Homeopath: Journal of the Society for Homeopaths*
http://www.homeopathy-soh.org/journal/

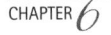

| TABLE 6-3 | Evidence-Based Summaries from Bandolier on the Efficacy of Homeopathy | |
| --- | --- | --- |
| SUMMARY TITLE | URL | REFERENCE |
| Arnica efficacy | http://www.jr2.ox.ac.uk/ bandolier/booth/ alternat/AT012.html | Ernst E, Pittler MH: Efficacy of homeopathic arnica: a systematic review of placebo-controlled clinical trials, *Arch Surg* 133:1187-1190, 1998. |
| Homeopathic remedies and quality | http://www.jr2.ox.ac.uk/ bandolier/booth/ alternat/homequal. html | Linde K and others: Impact of study quality on outcome in placebo-controlled trials of homeopathy, *J Clin Epidemiol* 52:631-636, 1999. Ernst E, Pittler MH: Re-analysis of previous meta-analysis of clinical trials of homeopathy, *J Clin Epidemiol* 53:1188, 2000. |
| Homeopathy for flu | http://www.jr2.ox.ac.uk/ bandolier/booth/ alternat/AT017.html | Vickers AJ, Smith C: Homeopathic *Oscillococcinum* for preventing and treating influenza and influenza-like syndromes (Cochrane review). In the *Cochrane Library*, issue 1, Oxford, 2000, Update Software. |
| Homeopathy for osteoarthritis | http://www.jr2.ox.ac.uk/ bandolier/booth/ alternat/homearth.html | Long L, Ernst E: Homeopathic remedies for the treatment of osteoarthritis: a systematic review, *Br Homeopath J* 90:37-43, 2001. |
| Homeopathy ineffective for headache | http://www.jr2.ox.ac.uk/ bandolier/band46/ b46-7.html | Walach H and others: Classical homeopathic treatment of chronic headaches, *Cephalalgia* 17:119-126, 1997. |
| Migraine prophylaxis with homeopathy | http://www.jr2.ox.ac.uk/ bandolier/booth/ alternat/AT015.html | Ernst E: Homeopathic prophylaxis of headaches and migraine: a systematic review, *J Pain Symptom Manage* 18(5):353-357, 1999. |
| Pollinosis and homeopathy | http://www.jr2.ox.ac.uk/ bandolier/booth/ alternat/AT013.html | Wiesenauer M, Ludtke R: A meta-analysis of the homeopathic treatment of pollinosis with *Galphimia glauca, Forsch Komplementarmed* 3:230-234, 1996. |
| Postoperative ileus | http://www.jr2.ox.ac.uk/ bandolier/band51/ b51-6.html | Barnes J, Resch K-L, Ernst E: Homeopathy for postoperative ileus? *J Clin Gastroenterol* 25:628-633, 1997. |

*Homeopathy Online*
http://www.lyghtforce.com/HomeopathyOnline/
*Simillimum: Journal of the Homeopathic Academy of Naturopathic Physicians*
http://www.healthy.net/library/journals/simillimum/

## Professional Organizations

**American Association of Naturopathic Physicians**
http://www.naturopathic.org/

American Institute of Homeopathy
http://www.homeopathyusa.org/
British Homeopathic Association
http://www.homeopathy.org
Council for Homeopathic Certification
http://www.homeopathicdirectory.com/old/index.htm
Homeopathic Academy of Naturopathic Physicians
http://www.healthy.net/pan/pa/homeopathic/hanp/index.html
National Board of Homeopathic Examiners
http://www.homeopathic.com/procare/procare.htm
National Center for Homeopathy
http://www.homeopathic.org/
North American Society of Homeopaths (NASH)
http://www.homeopathy.org/

### Internet Resources

Glasgow Homeopathic Hospital
http://www.homeoint.org/morrell/glasgow/index.htm
Homeopathic Educational Services
http://www.homeopathic.com/
Royal London Homeopathic Hospital NHS Trust
http://www.doh.gov.uk/hospitalactivity/index.htm

---

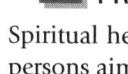 PRAYER, SPIRITUALITY, AND ENERGETIC THERAPIES

Spiritual healing is defined as "the systematic, purposeful intention by one or more persons aiming to help another person or living being or beings by means of focused attention, by touch, or by holding the hands near the other being, without application of physical, chemical, or conventional energetic means of intervention."[2]

Therapies included in spiritual healing range from faith healing practiced in churches to bioenergetic practices, *reiki*, Therapeutic Touch, and shamanism. Many of these approaches are based on the idea that the human body consists of energy fields that can be stimulated through various techniques to promote wellness. Themes include the awareness of self that extends beyond the physical body and the interconnectedness of humanity and divinity.

### Abstracts of Cochrane Collaboration Systematic Reviews

Abstracts of systematic reviews of the literature on spiritual healing are available from the Cochrane Collaboration at **<http://www.update-software.com/Cochrane/default.HTM>**.

### Evidence–Based Summaries from Bandolier

Table 6-4 lists evidence-based summaries from Bandolier describing the effects of spiritual healing on various conditions.

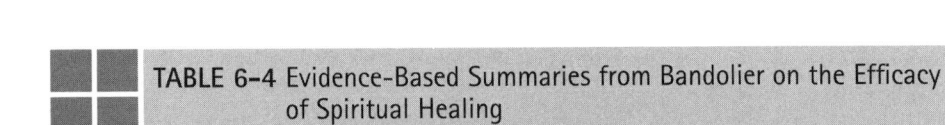

| TABLE 6-4 Evidence-Based Summaries from Bandolier on the Efficacy of Spiritual Healing | | |
|---|---|---|
| **TYPE OF THERAPY** | **URL** | **REFERENCE** |
| Power of prayer | http://www.jr2.ox.ac.uk/bandolier/band46/b46-6.html | Positive therapeutic effects of intercessionory prayer in a coronary care unit population, *South Med J* 81:826-829, 1988. |
| Therapeutic Touch | http://www.jr2.ox.ac.uk/bandolier/band51/b51-1.html | Cowl CT and others: Factors associated with fatalities and injuries from hot-air balloon crashes, *JAMA* 279:1011-1014, 1998. Kluger J: Mr Natural, *Time* May 19, 1997. p 44-51. Rosa L, Rosa E, Sarner L: A close look at Therapeutic Touch, *JAMA* 279:1005-1010, 1998. |

## Research Reports

The International Center for the Integration of Health and Spirituality (ICIHS) provides research reports on spiritual healing on its Web site at <**http://www.nihr.org/**>.

## Books

*Energy Medicine: The Scientific Basis of Bioenergy*
James Oschman and Candace Pert (foreword)
Churchill Livingstone, 2000
*Sacred Healing: The Curing Power of Energy and Spirituality*
Norman Shealy and Caroline Myss
Element Books, 1999
*Therapeutic Touch: Theory and Practice, ed. 2*
Jean Sayre-Adams and Stephen G. Wright
Harcourt International, 2001

## Journals

*International Journal of Aromatherapy*
http://www.harcourt-international.com/journals/ijar/
*Subtle Energies and Energy Medicine Journal*
http://www.issseem.org/journal.html

## Professional and Referral Organizations

**Healing Touch International**
http://www.healingtouch.net/index.shtml
**International Center for the Integration of Health and Spirituality**
http://www.nihr.org/

**International Society for the Study of Subtle Energies and Energy Medicine**
http://www.issseem.org/
**Nurse Healers-Professional Associates International (NH-PAI)**
http://www.therapeutic-touch.org/

## Internet Resources

**Energy Healing Systems: Reiki Internet Resources**
http://www.holisticmed.com/www/energy.html
**Healing Arts**
http://www.healing-arts-tt.com/Index.htm
**Therapeutic Touch**
http://bdenison.sbcusa.com/

## References

1. National Center for Homepathy, *http://www.homeopathic.org* (accessed 2/2/02).
2. Benor D: *Spiritual healing: does it work? Science says yes!* Southfield, MI, 1999, Vision Publications.

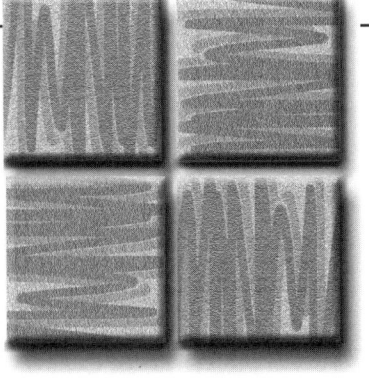

# CHAPTER 7

# Complementary and Alternative Medicine Resources for Health Professionals and Researchers

**Chapter Highlights**
Introduction
Physician Use and Interest in Complementary
    and Alternative Medicine
Guidelines and Consensus Statements
Special Reports and Articles Online
Federal Government Resources
Quality and Safety Sites
Research Resources
Nonprofit Organizations
Academic Research Organizations and Institutions
Products and Sites for Health Professionals
Conclusion

## ■ INTRODUCTION

In the previous chapters we have discussed the use and rationale for CAM among patients and health care consumers. As research into CAM continues, discussing these therapies will be increasingly important for the health care system and for health care providers. This discussion would not be complete without examining the quality Web-based information resources in CAM and the printed media and efficient tools for information management. With that in mind, this chapter is designed to provide a foundation for obtaining timely and accurate information on Internet-based and printed resources in CAM with an emphasis on profiling Web sites that provide the best available evidence and information for health care professionals.

##  PHYSICIAN USE AND INTEREST IN COMPLEMENTARY AND ALTERNATIVE MEDICINE

A recent review of 19 international surveys suggests that large numbers of conventional physicians are referring patients to CAM practitioners or are practicing some of the more prominent and well-known forms of CAM. Across the studies reviewed, acupuncture had the highest rate of physician referral (43%) among the five CAM therapies reviewed, followed by chiropractic (40%) and massage (21%). Conventional physicians practicing CAM varied from 9% for homeopathy to 19% for chiropractic and massage therapy.[1] Regarding perceived efficacy of CAM therapies by physicians in the review, the following values were observed: acupuncture (51%), chiropractic (53%), and massage (48%). Fewer physicians believed in the value of homeopathy (26%) and herbal approaches (13%).[2] Conditions for which physicians used or made referrals for these and other CAM therapies included chronic pain, back problems, psychological problems, headaches, and chronic illnesses. This review, however, showed great variations in the perceived efficacy of CAM therapies among physicians, which did not appear to be related to differences in the dates that the studies in the review were published or to the country in which the review was conducted. In many respects these variations in perceived efficacy may be due to the lack of accepted national and international standards regarding adequate scientific evidence for the inclusion of CAM into medical practice and referral. Furthermore, the incorporation of CAM is influenced by other factors, such as the availability of licensed or accredited practitioners, regional economics, and the regional cultural popularity of particular CAM therapies. Therefore, in an effort to support the safe and effective use of CAM therapies, this chapter indicates the best sources of Internet-based CAM interventions.

##  GUIDELINES AND CONSENSUS STATEMENTS

The following documents provide information on applying complementary and alternative medicine therapies to common health problems:

**Integration of Behavioral and Relaxation Approaches into the Treatment of Chronic Pain and Insomnia**
Technology Assessment Statements, October 16-18, 1995
http://odp.od.nih.gov/consensus/ta/017/017_intro.htm
**Consensus Statement on Acupuncture**
Vol. 15, No. 5, November 3-5,1997
http://odp.od.nih.gov/consensus/cons/107/107_intro.htm

## SPECIAL REPORTS AND ARTICLES ONLINE

The following resources offer insight into using complementary and alternative therapies:
*Alternative and Complementary Medicine Journal*
BioMed Central publishes systematic reviews and clinical trials of CAM therapies.
http://www.biomedcentral.com/1472-6882/

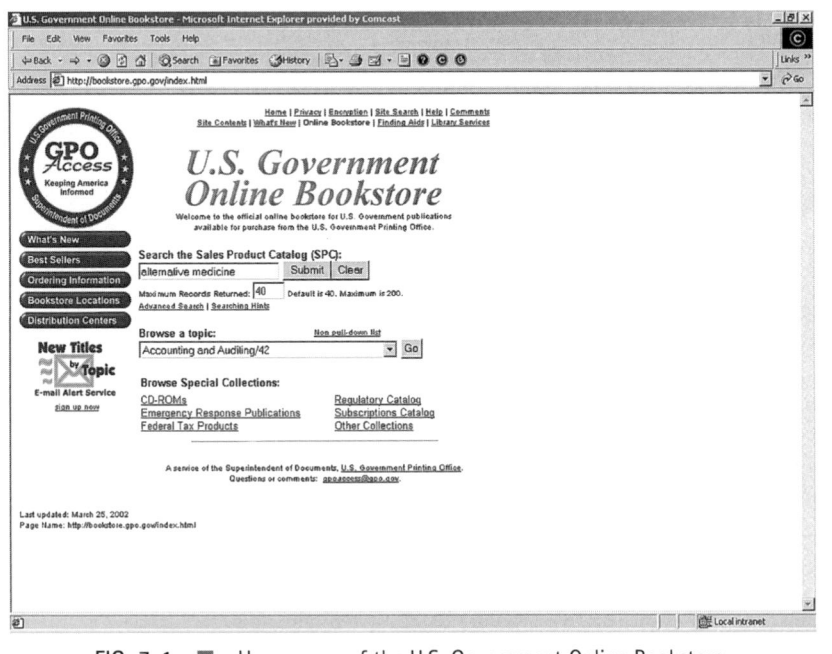

FIG. 7-1   ■   Home page of the U.S. Government Online Bookstore.

**Alternative Medicine: Expanding Medical Horizons**
This is a seminal report by the National Institutes of Health on alternative medical
  systems and practices in the United States (Fig. 7-1).
http://bookstore.gpo.gov/index.html.
**American Medical Association–published special reports**
These reports are available only to members of the assocation.
http://jama.ama-assn.org/issues/v280n18/toc.html
*Archives of General Psychiatry*
November 1998
http://archpsyc.ama-assn.org/
*Archives of Internal Medicine*
November 9, 1998
http://archinte.ama-assn.org/
*Archives of Neurology*
November 1998
http://archneur.ama-assn.org/
*British Medical Journal*
The Collected Resources in Complementary Medicine contains more than 60 articles
  on complementary medicine.
http://bmj.com/cgi/collection/complementary_medicine
*Complementary and Alternative Health Practices and Therapies*
York University Center for Health Studies
http://www.yorku.ca/research/ychs/html/publications.html

*Enhancing the Accountability of Alternative Medicine*
This text covers patient protection and the communication of scientific information.
New York, 1998, Milbank Memorial Fund
http://www.milbank.org/mraltmed.html
**Five-Year Strategic Plan: National Center for Complementary and Alternative Medicine**
http://nccam.nih.gov/about/plans/healthdisparities/appendices.htm
**Garlic: Effects on Cardiovascular Risks and Disease, Protective Effects against Cancer, and Clinical Adverse Effects**
http://www.ahrq.gov/clinic/garlicsum.htm
**Integrated Healthcare: A Way Forward for the Next Five Years?**
This article is published by the Foundation for Integrated Medicine (1997).
http://www.fimed.org/
*Journal of the American Medical Association*
November 11, 1998
http://jama.ama-assn.org/
**Milk Thistle: Effects on Liver Disease and Cirrhosis and Clinical Adverse Effects**
This evidence report details a systematic review summarizing clinical studies of milk thistle in humans.
http://www.ahrq.gov/clinic/milktsum.htm
**National HMO Survey of Alternative Care**
Landmark Health Care, Inc., 1999
http://www.landmarkhealthcare.com/
**A Systematic Review of the Quality of Homeopathic Clinical Trials**
Wayne B. Jonas and others
*BMC Complementary and Alternative Medicine* 1:12, 2001
http://www.biomedcentral.com/1472-6882/1/12/
**Systematic Review of the Use of Honey as a Wound Dressing**
Owen A. Moore and others
*BMC Complementary and Alternative Medicine* 1:2, 2001
http://www.biomedcentral.com/1472-6882/1/2/
**Systematic Reviews of Complementary Therapies: An Annotated Bibliography. Part 2. Herbal Medicine**
Klaus Linde and others
*BMC Complementary and Alternative Medicine* 1:5, 2001
http://www.biomedcentral.com/1472-6882/1/5/
**Systematic Reviews of Complementary Therapies: An Annotated Bibliography. Part 3. Homeopathy**
Klaus Linde and others
*BMC Complementary and Alternative Medicine* 1:4, 2001
http://www.biomedcentral.com/1472-6882/1/4/
**Systematic Reviews of Complementary Therapies: An Annotated Bibliography. Part 1. Acupuncture**
Klaus Linde and others

*BMC Complementary and Alternative Medicine* 1:3, 2001
http://www.biomedcentral.com/1472-6882/1/3/
**White House Commission Report on Complementary and Alternative Medicine Policy**
http://www.whccamp.hhs.gov/

---

 FEDERAL GOVERNMENT RESOURCES

### National Center for Complementary and Alternative Medicine
The National Center for Complementary and Alternative Medicine at the NIH has one of the most comprehensive CAM sites on the Web. Written with consumers in mind, the Web site also provides good general information for health care professionals. Established in 1998, the Web site reflects the growth of the center. Averaging more than 600,000 visits per month, the site includes links to NCCAM program areas, news and events, research grants, funding opportunities, and resources <http://www.nccam.nih.gov/> (Straus testimony, NCCR, 2001).

### CAM on PubMed
This collection of more than 220,000 citations is accessed through the PubMed database, which also includes MEDLINE. Sponsored by the NCBI, PubMed can be accessed at <http://www.ncbi.nlm.nih.gov/>.

### Combined Health Information Database
The federally supported Combined Health Information Database (CHID) is another service in which NCCAM participates and includes a variety of materials not available in other government databases. CHID aggregates health information for the public on numerous topics related to health and disease at <http://chid.nih.gov/> (Fig. 7-2).

### National Cancer Institute
Surveys indicate that, on average, over 30% of cancer sufferers use some form of CAM therapies during their illness.[3] In response, the NIH National Cancer Institute (NCI) Office of Cancer Complementary and Alternative Medicine (OCCAM) <http://www3.cancer. gov/occam/about.html> was established in October 1998 to coordinate and enhance the activities of the National Cancer Institute (NCI) in the arena of complementary and alternative medicine (CAM).

### Cancer Trials
An addition to the NCI Web site is the cancer trials site <http://www.nci.nih.gov/clinical_trials/>, which provides patients, health care professionals, and the public with information about ongoing NCI-sponsored trials, recent advances in cancer therapy, and resources related to cancer treatment (Fig. 7-3).

The Cancer Information Service (CIS) provides up-to-date cancer information to patients and their families, the public, and health care professionals in every state

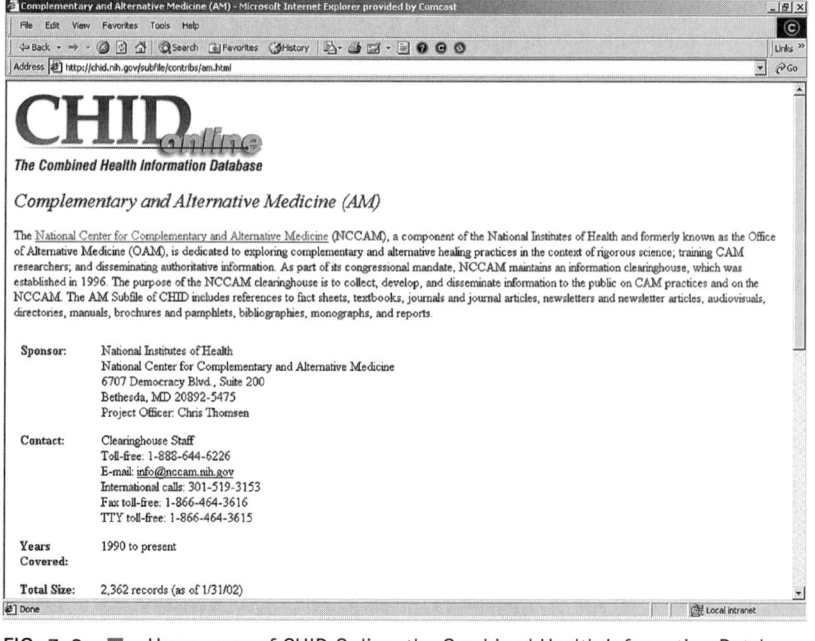

**FIG. 7–2** ■ Home page of CHID Online, the Combined Health Information Database.

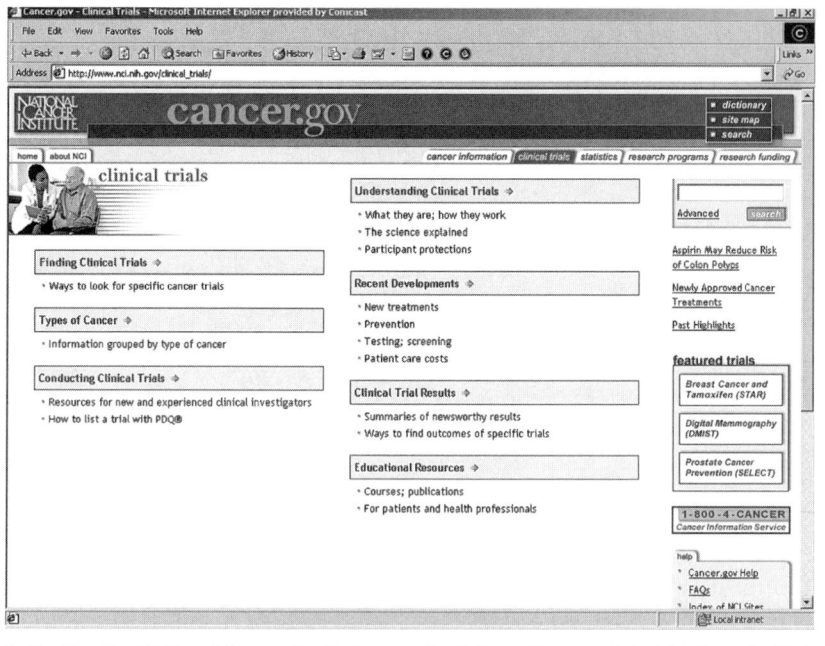

**FIG. 7–3** ■ The National Cancer Institute provides information on clinical trials on its Web site.

through 19 offices located in NCI-funded cancer centers and on the phone at 1-800-4-CANCER.

Through Physician Data Query (PDQ), NCI provides another source of information about NCI-sponsored trials at <**http://nci.nih.gov/**>.

## Additional Federal Government Resources

Various other government sites include content that relates to complementary and alternative therapies to the degree that their mandate includes some aspect of CAM oversight and informatics.

### White House Commission on Complementary and Alternative Medicine Policy

President Clinton formed WHCCAMP to make recommendations on public policy and legislation pertaining to complementary and alternative medicine. The Web site contains the full White House commission report and transcripts of town hall meetings at <**http://www.whccamp.hhs.gov/**> (Fig. 7-4).

### FirstGov

FirstGov is a massive federal database linked to federal documents located throughout government databases so that every federal document or page that appears on the

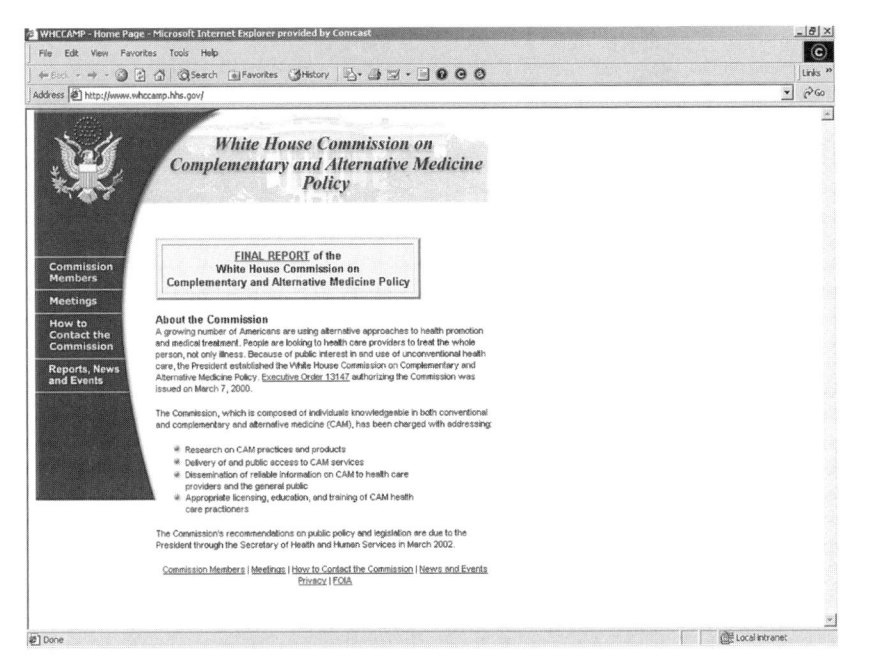

**FIG. 7-4** ■ Home page of the White House Commission on Complementary and Alternative Medicine Policy.

Web will be searched and posted by this site. All entries are rated by relevance. A search of *"alternative medicine"* produces links to 102,000 documents (accessed March 2001)—any Federal document or report that mentions alternative medicine. Fortunately, the entries include relevance ranking that indicates the percentage of content relevant to the topic. For example, documents from NCCAM are 99% relevant to the topic. The database, at **<http://www.firstgov.gov/>**, includes an exceptionally broad range of information.

### Office of Dietary Supplements, National Institutes of Health

The Office of Dietary Supplements (ODS) is involved in monitoring issues related to supplements and collects the results of research on dietary supplements, serving as a clearinghouse with databases and partnering with NIH and other federal institutions. The ODS provides a Web-searchable database, International Bibliographic Information on Dietary Supplements, which contains more than 400,000 bibliographic citations and abstracts, primarily on dietary supplements. The agency also provides another database, Computer Access to Research on Dietary Supplements (CARDS). The databases are available at **<http://dietary-supplements.info.nih.gov/>**.

 ## QUALITY AND SAFETY SITES

### Food and Drug Administration

The FDA regulates dietary supplements under a different set of regulations than those covering conventional foods and drug products (prescription and over-the-counter drugs). Under the Dietary Supplement Health and Education Act of 1994 (DSHEA), the dietary supplement manufacturer is responsible for ensuring that a dietary supplement is safe before it is marketed. FDA is responsible for taking action against any unsafe dietary supplement product after it reaches the market. Generally, manufacturers do not need to register with the FDA or get FDA approval before producing or selling dietary supplements. Manufacturers must make sure that product label information is truthful and not misleading. The postmarketing responsibilities of the FDA include monitoring safety (for example, voluntary dietary supplement adverse event reporting) and product information such as labeling, claims, package inserts, and accompanying literature. The FDA Web site is **<http://www.fda.gov/>**.

The Food and Drug Administration food safety site is **<http://www.cfsan.fda.gov/>**.

### Dietary Supplements/Food Labeling Electronic Newsletter

For an electronic newletter on dietary supplements and food labeling regulations, see **<http://vm.cfsan.fda.gov/~dms/fda-dsfl.html>**.

### Centers for Disease Control and Prevention

In the area of CAM, the CDC has taken a role in monitoring herbal supplements and also has analyzed data on nutritional supplements. Although the CDC Web site does not post pages dedicated specifically to alternative medicine, a subject search yielded

40 documents, primarily reports in portable document format files. All entries are ranked by relevance to the topic. Of the first 20 documents, 19 were published within the past 15 months. The CDC site, at <**http://www.cdc.gov/**>, also provides excellent, up-to-date information regarding infectious disease, outbreaks, and epidemiology.

### Federal Trade Commission

The FTC protects consumers by pursuing organizations that fraudulently market products and services on the Web. Recent enforcement actions have been taken and are currently under way. Such information is available at <**http://www.ftc.gov/opa/2001/06/cureall.htm**>.

### Canadian Natural Health Products Directorate

The new Canadian Natural Health Products Directorate will have the authority to approve natural health products for the Canadian market, ensuring Canadian consumers have safe natural health products. The Web site is <**http://www.hc-sc.gc.ca/hpb/onhp/welcome_e.html**>.

### Health Protection Branch, Canada

The Health Protection Branch in Canada regulates and controls medical devices, product safety, drugs, and so on. The Web site is <**http://www.hc-sc.gc.ca/hpb/**>.

 RESEARCH RESOURCES

NCCAM funds and monitors more CAM research than any other institution in the United States. The level of appropriation for NCCAM has been increased twice to a budget of $113 million for the year 2003. As a result of partnering with other sections of the NIH, NCCAM has achieved aggregate funding totaling roughly $200 million for 2002. Table 7-1 provides list of clinical trials that currently are recruiting subjects.

ClinicalTrials.gov provides a complete listing of all CAM trials sponsored by the NIH. For a complete listing of clinical studies in CAM, one may search under the keyword *"alternative medicine."* As of April 2002, 147 clinical trials were listed at <**http://www.clinicaltrials.gov/**>.

In addition to funding individual clinical trials, NCCAM has funded or provided additional funding for 15 research centers in the United States (Table 7-2). Each program concentrates on prevention and treatment of at least one major disease condition or on the health issue of a particular population. These centers in turn have the ability to fund pilot studies known as development-of-feasibility projects. Given the focus of each of these centers, they are in a position to conduct, assess, and stimulate research within their field of study. Quite a few research organizations now are focused on complementary medicine; most often these are medical schools that are involved in performing research and teaching medical students. A number of these organizations also have developed integrative clinics for treating patients. Some institutions, such as the University of Maryland, include a focus on informatics.

**TABLE 7-1** National Center for Complementary and Alternative Medicine Clinical Trials Currently Recruiting Volunteers*

| PHASE III CLINICAL TRIALS | STATUS | COSPONSORING SECTIONS OF THE NIH | TARGET ENROLLMENT | CLINICALTRIALS.GOV URL |
|---|---|---|---|---|
| Acupuncture for osteoarthritis pain | Enrolling subjects | NIAMS† | 570 | http://clinicaltrials.gov/ct/gui/c/w1r/show/NCT00010946?order=2&ServSessionIdzone_ct=mhxnx862t1 |
| EDTA chelation therapy for treating coronary artery disease | Under review | NHLBI | 1600 (estimated) | Not available |
| Ginkgo biloba for preventing dementia | Enrolling subjects | NIA, NHLBI, NINDS | 3000-3500 | http://clinicaltrials.gov/ct/gui/c/w1r/show/NCT00029679?order=4&ServSessionIdzone_ct=mhxnx862t1 |
| Glucosamine/chondroitin for treating osteoarthritis | Enrolling subjects | NIAMS | 1588 | http://clinicaltrials.gov/ct/gui/c/w1r/show/NCT00010790?order=1&ServSessionIdzone_ct=mhxnx862t1 |
| Hypericum perforatum for treating minor depression | Awarded | NIMH, ODS | 300 (minimum) | Not available |
| Saw palmetto and Pygeum africanum for preventing progression of benign prostatic hypertrophy | Announced | NIDDK, ODS | 3000 (estimated) | Not available |
| Shark cartilage as adjunct therapy for lung cancer | Enrolling subjects | NCI | 756 | http://clinicaltrials.gov/ct/gui/c/w1r/show/NCT00005838?order=1&ServSessionIdzone_ct=mhxnx862t1 |
| Vitamin E/selenium for treating prostate cancer | Enrolling subjects | NCI | 32,400 | http://clinicaltrials.gov/ct/gui/c/w1r/show/NCT00006392?order=3&ServSessionIdzone_ct=mhxnx862t1 |

*From Straus S: Congressional testimony, 2002.

†NIAMS, National Institute of Arthritis and Musculoskeletal and Skin Diseases; NHLBI, National Heart, Lung, and Blood Institute; NIA, National Institute on Aging; NINDS, National Institute of Neurological Disorders and Stroke; NIMH, National Institute of Mental Health; NIDDK, National Institute of Diabetes and Digestive and Kidney Diseases.

**TABLE 7-2** Research Centers Funded by the National Center for Complementary and Alternative Medicine

| SPECIALTY | PRINCIPAL INVESTIGATOR AND INSTITUTION | URL |
|---|---|---|
| Addictions | Thomas J. Kiresuk, Ph.D.<br>Center for Addiction and Alternative<br>  Medicine Research<br>Minneapolis Medical Research Foundation<br>914 South Eighth Street, Suite D917<br>Minneapolis, MN 55404 | http://www.mmrfweb.org/<br>research/addicton&alt_<br>med/index.html |
| Aging and<br>  women's health | Fredi Kronenberg, Ph.D.<br>Center for CAM Research in Aging and<br>  Women's Health<br>Columbia University<br>College of Physicians and Surgeons<br>630 West 168th Street<br>New York, NY 10032 | http://www.rosenthal.hs.<br>columbia.edu/Aging.<br>html |
| Arthritis | Brian M. Berman, M.D.<br>Center for Alternative Medicine Research<br>  on Arthritis<br>University of Maryland School of Medicine<br>Center for Integrative Medicine<br>2200 Kernan Drive<br>Baltimore, MD 21207-6693 | http://www.compmed.<br>umm.edu |
| Botanicals | Connie M. Weaver, Ph.D.<br>Botanical Center for Age-Related Diseases<br>Purdue University, West Lafayette<br>Division of Sponsored Programs<br>West Lafayette, IN 47907-1021 | http://fn.cfs.purdue.<br>edu/bot |
| | David Heber, M.D., Ph.D.<br>UCLA Center for Dietary Supplements<br>  Research: Botanicals<br>University of California at Los Angeles<br>10945 Le Conte Avenue, Suite 1401<br>Box 951406<br>Los Angeles, CA 90095-1406 | No URL available |
| | Barbara N. Timmermann, Ph.D.<br>Arizona Center for Phytomedicine Research<br>University of Arizona College of Pharmacy<br>1703 East Mabel<br>P.O. Box 210207<br>Tucson, AZ 85721-0207 | http://acprx.pharmacy.<br>arizona.edu/ |
| Cancer | Adrian S. Dobs, M.D.<br>Johns Hopkins Center for Cancer<br>  Complementary Medicine<br>Johns Hopkins University<br>720 Rutland Avenue<br>Baltimore, MD 21205 | http://www.hopkins-cam.<br>org/ |

*Continued*

| SPECIALTY | PRINCIPAL INVESTIGATOR AND INSTITUTION | URL |
|---|---|---|
| Cancer—cont'd | Stephen R. Thom, M.D., Ph.D.<br>Secialized Center of Research in Hyperbaric<br>　Oxygen Therapy<br>University of Pennsylvania<br>133 South 36th Street<br>Research Services, Mezzanine<br>Philadelphia, PA 19104-3246 | http://www.uphs.upenn.<br>edu/ifem/scor_in_<br>hyperbaric_oxygen_<br>therap.htm |
| Cardiovascular<br>disease<br>and aging<br>in African-<br>Americans | Robert H. Schneider, M.D.<br>Center for Natural Medicine and Prevention<br>Maharishi University of Management<br>504 North 4th Street, Suite 207<br>Fairfield, IA 52557 | http://www.mum.edu/<br>CNMP |
| Cardiovascular<br>diseases | Steven F. Bolling, M.D.<br>Center for Complementary and Alternative<br>　Medicine Research in CVD<br>Adult Cardiac Surgery/Thoracic<br>　Transplantation<br>The University of Michigan Taubman Health<br>　Care Center<br>715 Huron Street, Suite 1W<br>Ann Arbor, MI 48109 | http://www.med.umich.<br>edu/camrc/index.html |
| Chiropractic | William C. Meeker, D.C., M.P.H.<br>Consortial Center for Chiropractic Research<br>Palmer Center for Chiropractic Research<br>741 Brady Street<br>Davenport, IA 52803 | http://www.palmer.edu |
| Craniofacial<br>disorders | B. Alexander White, D.D.S.<br>Center for Health Research<br>Kaiser Foundation Hospitals<br>3800 North Interstate Avenue<br>Portland, OR 97227-1110 | No URL available |
| Neurodegenerative<br>diseases | Mahlon R. Delong, M.D.<br>Center for CAM in Neurodegenerative<br>　Diseases<br>Department of Neurology<br>Emory University School of Medicine<br>1639 Pierce Drive<br>Atlanta, GA 30322 | http://www.emory.edu/<br>WHSC/MED/<br>NEUROLOGY/<br>CAM/index.html |
| Neurological<br>disorders | Barry S. Oken, M.D.<br>Oregon Center for Complementary and<br>　Alternative Medicine in Neurological<br>　Disorders<br>Oregon Health Sciences University<br>3181 SW Sam Jackson Park Road<br>Portland, OR 97201 | http://www.ohsu.edu/<br>orccamind/ |

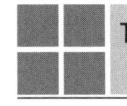

| SPECIALTY | PRINCIPAL INVESTIGATOR AND INSTITUTION | URL |
|-----------|----------------------------------------|-----|
| | **TABLE 7-2** Research Centers Funded by the National Center for Complementary and Alternative Medicine—cont'd | |
| Pediatrics | Fayez K. Ghishan, M.D., D.C.H.<br>University of Arizona Health Sciences Center<br>Department of Pediatrics<br>1501 North Campbell Avenue<br>P.O. Box 245073<br>Tucson, AZ 85724-5073 | No URL available |

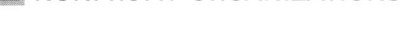

## NONPROFIT ORGANIZATIONS

### Cochrane Collaboration Complementary Medicine Field

Funding of the Cochrane Complementary Medicine Field was awarded in 1996 through a supplemental grant to the University of Maryland Program of Complementary Medicine[4] <http://www.compmed.umm.edu/>. In the first phase of work, a high priority was placed on building the infrastructure necessary to make the Complementary Medicine (CM) Field a functioning entity. In the brief time that the CM Field has been functioning, a great deal of effort has been focused on laying the groundwork for reviews by constructing a database of all the known randomized controlled trials (RCTs) that pertain to complementary medicine, published or unpublished, in any language. Many of the challenges and difficulties of finding relevant studies, some unique to CM, are highlighted in an article that appeared in *JAMA* in November 1998.[5] To date, approximately 5800 CM RCTs and more than 230 systematic reviews have been identified. All RCTs in the specialized database are periodically uploaded to the main database of the Cochrane Collaboration, known as CENTRAL, which houses all the known randomized controlled trials for all of medicine. The CENTRAL registry is searchable by anyone with access to the Cochrane Library <http://www.update-software.com/cochrane/>. To locate additional trials, members of the CM Field hand search more than 30 high-priority journals on an ongoing basis. The significance of the CM field is that it consolidates and aggregates international efforts in the collection, evaluation, and dissemination of research in complementary and alternative therapies.

### Cochrane Collaboration Consumer Network

The Cochrane Collaboration Consumer Network site contains a range of health care and other information to help individuals understand health care research. The site also is a resource for consumers and others who want to become involved in the collaboration or other health research activities. In addition, the Consumer Network contains more than 28 consumer summaries of Cochrane reviews in CAM at <http://www.cochraneconsumer.com/index.asp?SHOW> (Fig. 7-5).

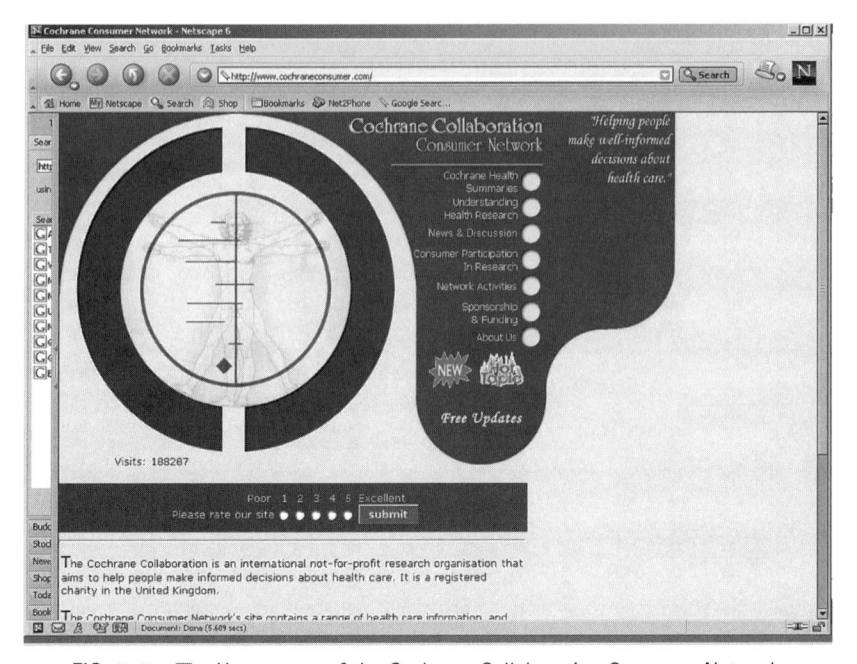

**FIG. 7-5** 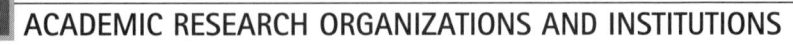 Home page of the Cochrane Collaboration Consumer Network.

### Bandolier (United Kingdom) Complementary and Alternative Therapies

The Bandolier site is intended to gather the best evidence available about complementary and alternative therapies (CATs) for the public and professionals, to update it as more or better evidence becomes available, and to have it accessible over the Internet at <http://www.jr2.ox.ac.uk/Bandolier/booth/booths/altmed.html>.

### Organising Medical Networked Information

OMNI is a gateway to evaluated, quality Internet resources in health and medicine, aimed at students, researchers, academics, and practitioners in the health and medical sciences at <http://omni.ac.uk/>.

### Alternative Medicine Foundation

The Alternative Medicine Foundation is a nonprofit 501(c)(3) organization founded in March 1998 to provide responsible and reliable information about alternative medicine to the public and health professionals. The Web site is <http://www. amfoundation.org>.

## ACADEMIC RESEARCH ORGANIZATIONS AND INSTITUTIONS

The following organizations and institutions conduct research into complementary and alternative therapies.

**Bastyr University**
Bastyr is a leading research center in natural health sciences.
http://www.bastyr.edu/
**Beth Israel Medical Center, New York**
Continuum Center for Health and Healing
The center provides fully integrative care, using safe and effective conventional and
    complementary therapies.
http://www.healthandhealingny.org/
**Center for Complementary Medicine Research**
This leading German CAM research organization is dedicated to research education
    and patient care.
http://www.lrz-muenchen.de/~ZentrumfuerNaturheilkunde/
**Exeter University**
The university is a research organization and publisher of *FACT: Focus on Alternative
    and Complementary Therapies,* a review journal that aims to present the evidence on
    complementary medicine in an analytical and impartial manner.
http://www.ex.ac.uk/
**Harvard University**
Center for Alternative Medicine Research and Education
The center is a leading research organization in CAM. The center sponsors annual
    conferences.
http://www.bidmc.harvard.edu/medicine/camr
**Jefferson University**
Center for Integrative Medicine
The Center for Integrative Medicine located at the Thomas Jefferson University
    Hospital and Thomas Jefferson University is conducting NIH-funded research on
    CAM therapies and quality of life for cancer patients.
http://www.jeffersonhospital.org/e3front.dll?durki=6953&site=347&return=8842
**Minneapolis Medical Research Foundation**
Center for Addiction and Alternative Medicine Research (CAAMR)
http://www.mmrfweb.org/research/addiction&alt_med/index.html
**Palmer Center for Chiropractic Research**
Consortial Center for Chiropractic Research
http://www.palmer.edu
**Research Council for Complementary Medicine (RCCM)**
This research organization is based in the United Kingdom and is the originator of
    the CISCOM database.
http://www.rccm.org.uk/
**Stanford University**
Center for Research in Disease Prevention
The Complementary and Alternative Medicine Program at Stanford (CAMPS)
The center is researching the topic of successful aging.
http://camps.stanford.edu/

**Tzu Chi Foundation**
The activities of this Canadian organization include clinical treatment programs, research, education, and information.
http://www.tzuchi.org/
**University of California, Irvine**
Susan Samueli Center for Complementary and Alternative Medicine
http://www.ucihs.uci.edu/com/samueli/
**University of California, San Francisco**
Osher Center for Integrative Medicine
http://www.ucsf.edu/ocim/
**University of Minnesota**
Center for Spirituality and Healing
The Center for Spirituality and Healing at the University of Minnesota was awarded a 5-year grant from the National Institutes of Health National Center for Complementary and Alternative Medicine (NCCAM). The grant supports the development and integration of complementary and alternative medicine (CAM) educational resources and programs in the curricula of the University's schools and colleges of Medicine, Nursing, and Pharmacy.
http://www.csh.umn.edu/
**University of Texas**
M.D. Anderson Cancer Center Complementary Therapy Reviews
Extensive list of evidence-based summaries conducted on complementary therapies used in the treatment of cancer.
http://www.mdanderson.org/departments/cimer/dIndex.cfm?pn=6EB86A59-EBD9-11D4-810100508B603A14

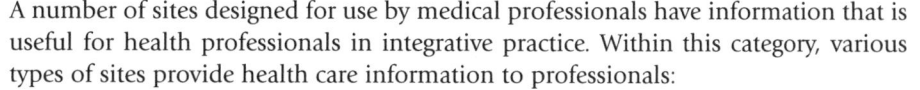 **PRODUCTS AND SITES FOR HEALTH PROFESSIONALS**

A number of sites designed for use by medical professionals have information that is useful for health professionals in integrative practice. Within this category, various types of sites provide health care information to professionals:

- Professional sites available by subscription
- Nonprofit consortia, such as the Cochrane Library, available by subscription
- Sites that are posted and maintained by associations, organizations, and institutions

Professional sites such as Medscape, MD Consult, and WebMD tend to be oriented toward mainstream physicians who are becoming involved in or have an interest in complementary therapies or integrative practice. Some sites, such as WebMD, also include and organize information that is intended for consumers. Finding good information that is free on the professional sites can be difficult. Currently the federal government is a primary source of free quality information through the NCCAM site and via federal resources including CAM on PubMed, ClinicalTrials.gov, and MEDLINEplus. Of the fee-access sites, the best are specific, well referenced, and focused on quality, safety, and efficacy. That said, even subscription-based information varies in its approach to integrative content. The CAM field is developing and will be defined differently by content providers. Such differences are reflected in the choice of information, type of content, and the degree of integration reflected in the protocol and guidelines. Resources intended for health care professionals include those discussed in the following sections.

## Cochrane Library

The Cochrane Collaboration was established in October of 1993 and aims to provide reliable, high-quality, evidence-based information by preparing, maintaining, and promoting the conduct and accessibility of systematic reviews of all available evidence regarding the benefits and risks of health care.[6,7] The cornerstone of this process is the systematic review. Currently in the Cochrane Library alone are more than 1000 published systematic reviews and several hundred protocols. To date, the Cochrane Library contains more than 5700 trials and 80 systematic reviews in CAM with an additional 60 systematic reviews now in progress. The Web site is **<http://www.cochranelibrary.com/clibhome/clib.htm>**.

## MD Consult

MD Consult is a fee-based service published by Elsevier Science that is geared to the needs of the physician. Readers can obtain and search full-text journal articles and medical textbooks, review clinical guidelines, and obtain detailed information. Searching for CAM information on MD Consult reveals a wealth of material, including reference books, journal articles, practice guidelines, news and reports, and patient handouts. Among the fee-based sites, MD Consult provides the most comprehensive peer-reviewed information on complementary or integrative medicine at **<http://home.mdconsult.com>**.

## Healthnotes

Healthnotes develops and distributes fully referenced, scientific, and balanced information on CAM. Gathered from scientific studies, the information is incorporated into a variety of print and electronic products, including the *Healthnotes Review of Complementary and Integrative Medicine*, the *Clinical Essentials Series for Healthcare Professionals*, and Healthnotes Online. The Web site is **<http://www.healthnotes.com/index.cfm>**.

## WebMD/Medscape

WebMD/Medscape is a comprehensive site offering Internet-based medical information for consumers and professionals. The site **<http://www.medscape.com/>** includes extensive content on alternative and complementary medicine resources for patients. Registration is required.

## Integrative Medicine Communications

Integrative Medicine Communications offers an extensive database on the clinical use of nutraceuticals, herbals, and alternative therapies in patient care. The information is based on medical literature and includes the German Commission E monographs on botanicals. This content also is updateable in notebook form (Access) or through newsletters such as the *Integrative Medicine Consult*. The Web site is <http://www.onemedicine.com/>.

## American WholeHealth

American WholeHealth is an Internet-enabled integrative medicine company, which offers services on conventional medicine and alternative therapies for consumers, practitioners, health plans, and employees. The Web site is **<http://www.american wholehealth.com/>.**

## Natural Medicines Comprehensive Database

The Natural Medicines Comprehensive Database is a database on natural products that is navigated easily and permits subscribers to ask the panel of experts questions such as which specific formulations of *Ginkgo biloba* actually were used in the clinical trials that established its efficacy for Alzheimer's disease and receive a prompt reply. This resource is regularly updated at **<http://www.naturaldatabase.com/>.**

## ConsumerLab.com

ConsumerLab.com is a laboratory that provides test results evaluating the quality of vitamin and herbal products. The reviews are available by subscription. The company description states, "ConsumerLab.com, LLC ('CL') provides independent test results and information to help consumers and healthcare professionals evaluate health, wellness, and nutrition products." The Web site is **<http://www.consumerlab.com>.**

## Books

*ABC of Complementary Medicine*
R. Zollman and A. Vickers
BMJ Books, 2000
*Acupressure: Clinical Applications in Musculo-Skeletal Conditions*
John R. Cross and James L. Oschman, 2001
*Acupuncture Efficacy: A Compendium of Controlled Clinical Studies*
Stephen Birch and Richard Hammerschlag
National Academy of Acupuncture and Oriental Medicine, 1996
*Acupuncture Energetics: A Clinical Approach for Physicians*
Joseph M. Helms
Medical Acupuncture, 1996
*Acupuncture, Trigger Points, and Musculoskeletal Pain*
P.F. Baldry
Churchill Livingstone, 1993
Musculoskeletal or myofascial pain often is a neglected area of study and is covered in relation to its successful treatment by acupuncture.
*Acupuncture: A Comprehensive Text*
Dan Bensky and John O'Connor, 1981

*The Alternative Medicine Handbook: The Complete Reference Guide to Alternative and Complementary Therapies*
Barrie R. Cassileth
W.W. Norton, 1998
*Alternative Medicine: What Works*
Adraine Fugh-Berman
William & Wilkins, 1997
*The Arthritis Foundation's Guide to Alternative Therapies*
Judith Horstman and William J. Arnold
Harper Collins College, 1999
*Basics of Acupuncture*
Gabriel Stux and Bruce Pomerantz
Springer Verlag, 1998
*The Best Alternative Medicine: What Works? What Does Not?*
Kenneth R. Pelletier
Simon Schuster, 2000
*Botanical Influences on Illness*
Melvin R. Werbach and Michael T. Murray
Third Line Press, 2000
*Chinese Acupuncture and Moxibustion*
Cheng Xin-nong
China Books & Periodicals, April 2000
*Clinical Acupuncture*
Gabriel Stux, R. Hammershlag, and B.M. Berman
Churchill Livingstone, 2000
*Clinical Acupuncture: Scientific Basis*
Gabriel Stux
Springer Verlag, 2000
*Clinical Research: Methodology for Complementary Therapies*
George T. Lewith and David Aldridge, editors
Hodder & Stroughton, 1987
*Clinician's Complete Reference to Complementary & Alternative Medicine*
Donald Novey
Mosby, 2000
*Color Atlas of Acupuncture: Body Points, Ear Points, Trigger Points*
Hans-Ulrich Hecker and others
Thieme Medical Publishers, 2001
*Complementary and Alternative Medicine: Legal Boundaries and Regulatory Perspectives*
Michael H. Cohen
John Hopkins University Press, 1998
*Complementary Medicine: An Integrated Approach*
George Lewith and Julian Kenyon
Oxford University Press, 1997

*Contemporary Chinese Medicine and Acupuncture*
Claire Cassidy, editor
Churchill Livingstone, 2001
*The Cross Name Index to Medicinal Plants, vol. 4, Plants in Indian Medicine A-Z*
Anthony R. Torkelson
CRC Press, 1999
*Energy Medicine: The Scientific Basis of Bioenergy*
James Oschman and Candace Pert (foreword)
Churchill Livingstone, 2000
*Essentials of Complementary and Alternative Medicine*
Wayne B. Jonas and Jeffrey S. Levin
Lippincott Williams & Wilkins, 1999
*Foundations of Chinese Medicine*
Giovanni Maciocia
Churchill Livingstone, 1997
*Foundations of Nutritional Medicine: A Sourcebook of Clinical Research*
Melvin R. Werbach
Third Line Press, 1997
*The Handbook of Alternative and Complementary Medicine*
Stephen Fulder
Oxford University Press, 1996
*Herbal Medicine: Expanded Commission E Monographs*
M. Blumenthal, A. Goldberg, and J. Newton Brinckmann
Integrative Medicine Communications, 2000
*Medical Acupuncture*
J. Filshie and A. White
Churchill Livingstone, 1997
*Medical Massage*
Ross Turchaninov and Connie A. Cox
Aesculapius Books, 1998
*Professional's Handbook of Complementary and Alternative Medicines*
Charles W. Fetrow and Juan R. Avila
Springhouse, 1999
*Sacred Healing: The Curing Power of Energy and Spirituality*
Norman Shealy and Caroline Myss
Element Books, 1999
*Scientific Basis of Acupuncture*
Gabriel Stux and others, editors
Springer Verlag, 2000
*Therapeutic Touch: Theory and Practice, ed. 2*
Jean Sayre-Adams and Stephen G. Wright
Harcourt International, 2001
*The Web That Has No Weaver*
Ted Kaptchuck
Contemporary Books, 2000

## Journals

*Advances in Mind-Body Medicine*
http://www.harcourt-international.com/journals/ambm/
*Aesclepian Chronicles*
http://www.forthrt.com/%7Echronicl/homepage.html
*Alternative Medicine Alert*
http://www.altmednet.com/
*Alternative Medicine Digest*
http://www.alternativemedicine.com/
*Alternative Medicine Magazine*
http://nbaf.com/subscriptions/he/am.html
*Alternative Medicine Review*
http://www.thorne.com/altmedrev/index.html
*Alternative Therapies in Health and Medicine*
http://www.alternative-therapies.com/
*American Journal of Clinical Hypnosis*
http://www.asch.net/ajch.htm
*Australian Journal of Clinical & Experimental Hypnosis*
http://www.ozhypnosis.com.au
*Australian Traditional-Medicine Society*
http://www.atms.com.au/
**BioMed Central**
For journals, see http://www.biomedcentral.com
**British Acupuncture Council**
For resources, see http://www.acupuncture.org.uk/
*British Homeopathic Journal*
http://www.homeocases.org/article.asp
*British Medical Journal* Collected Resources
http://www.bmj.com/
*Canadian Journal of Herbalism*
http://www.herbalists.on.ca/journal/
*Chinese Journal of Digestive Diseases*
http://www.blackwell-science.com/%7Ecgilib/jnlpage.bin?Journal=cdd&File=
    cdd&Page=aims
*Clinical Acupuncture and Oriental Medicine*
http://www.harcourt-international.com/journals/caom/default.cfm
*Complementary Therapies in Medicine*
http://www.harcourt-international.com/journals/ctim/
*Complementary Therapies in Nursing & Midwifery*
http://www.harcourt-international.com/journals/ctnm/
*European Journal of Clinical Hypnosis*
http://www.ejch.com/
*European Journal of Herbal Medicine*
http://www.nimh.btinternet.co.uk/ejhm/

*European Journal of Oriental Medicine*
http://www.ejom.co.uk/
*Fitoterapia*
http://www.elsevier.nl/locate/fitote
*Focus on Alternative and Complementary Therapies*
http://www.ex.ac.uk/FACT/index.htm
*Forschende Komplementärmedizin*
http://www.karger.com/journals/fkm/fkm_jh.htm
*Homeopathy Today*
http://www.homeopathic.org/HTnew.htm
*International Journal of Aromatherapy*
http://www.harcourt-international.com/journals/ijar/
*International Journal of Clinical and Experimental Hypnosis*
http://sunsite.utk.edu/IJCEH/
*Journal of Alternative & Complementary Medicine*
http://www.liebertpub.com/ACM/default1.asp
*Journal of Bodywork & Movement Therapies*
http://www.harcourt-international.com/journals/jbmt/
*Journal of Ethnopharmacology*
http://www.elsevier.nl/inca/publications/store/5/0/6/0/3/5/
*Journal of Interprofessional Care*
http://www.staff.city.ac.uk/s.reeves-1/
*Journal of Manipulative and Physiological Therapeutics*
http://www.harcourthealth.com/scripts/om.dll/serve?action=searchDB&searchDB
    for=home&id=pt
*Journal of the American Institute of Homeopathy*
http://www.homeopathyusa.org/journal/
*Manual Therapy*
http://www.harcourt-international.com/journals/math/
*Medical Herbalism*
http://medherb.com/MHHOME.SHTML
*Midwifery*
http://www.harcourt-international.com/journals/midw/
*Nordic Journal of Music Therapy*
http://www.hisf.no/njmt/
*Pharmaceutical Biology*
http://www.szp.swets.nl/szp/journals/pb.htm
*Phytomedicine*
http://www.urbanfischer.de/journals/frame_template.htm?/journals/phytomed/
    phytmed.htm
*Phytomedicine*
http://www.nhaa.org.au/journal.html
*Research in Complementary and Classical Natural Medicine*
http://www.karger.ch/journals/fkm/fkm_jh.htm

*Scientific Review of Alternative Medicine*
http://primarycare.medscape.com/Prometheus/SRAM/public/SRAM-journal.html
*Simillimum*
http://www.urbanfischer.de/journals/frame_template.htm?/journals/phytomed/
  phytmed.htm

## News Sites

The value of news for researchers is its topical nature, reporting on what is being published in the scientific and medical literature. News sites also may report on use, new
developments, and trends in the field. To stay abreast of complementary medicine,
one will find it important to scan topical media sources—including newspapers,
magazines, newsletters, and the Web—for new therapies and new research. Just because a controlled clinical trial has not been done does not represent proof that a
therapy does or does not work. Epidemiological data and trends are other types of information available from news sources. In the context of how one gathers and synthesizes information, topical content has relevance. The following are Web sites providing news on complementary and alternative medicine.

**ABC NEWS.com: Health & Living News Index**
http://www.abcnews.com/sections/Living/
**Alternative Health News Online**
http://www.altmedicine.com/FrameSet.asp
**CNN Daily Updates on Health Topics**
http://www.medscape.com/Home/Topics/multispecialty/multispecialty.html
**Health Watch Web site**
http://www.trufax.org/menu/health1.html
**HealthWell Natural News**
http://www.healthwell.com/news/index.cfm
**Medscape Medical Research News**
http://www.medscape.com/medscapetodayhome
**Natural Health Line**
http://www.naturalhealthvillage.com/
*New York Times* **Daily Health News: Your Health Daily**
http://yourhealthdaily.com/
**Reuters Health Information Services, Inc.**
http://www.reutershealth.com/
**Science Daily News**
http://www.sciencedaily.com/index.htm
*USA Today* **Health**
http://www.usatoday.com/life/health/health.htm

## Newsletters

The Internet meets an important need in providing and disseminating information
on alternative therapies. Links between the publishing industry and the Internet reflect the breadth of the technology transfer that is taking place through books and
content that include medical textbooks, texts used in the training of CAM professionals, quality CAM journals, full-text journal articles available online, quality trade

**TABLE 7-3** Newsletters on Complementary and Alternative Medicine

| NEWSLETTER | URL |
|---|---|
| *Bandolier*<br>Andrew Moore, executive editor<br>National Health Service Research and Development Directorate<br>Contains bullet points (hence Bandolier) of evidence-based medicine and covers CM topics. | http://www.jr2.ox.ac.uk/Bandolier/ |
| *Complementary Medicine Field Newsletter*<br>Cochrane Collaboration<br>Karen Soeken, executive editor<br>Details activities and progress of the Cochrane Complementary Medicine Field. | http://www.compmed.umm.edu/<br>Cochrane/Newsletters/Spring2002. |
| *HerbalGram*<br>Herb Research Foundation | http://www.herbs.org/pubHG.html |
| *HerbClip*<br>Herb Research Foundation | http://www.herbs.org/green aper.html |
| *Integrative Medicine Consult*<br>Leonard Wisneski, editor<br>Provides impartial, up-to-date, science-based information about alternative therapies and botanical medicines in short summaries and discussions tailored to the needs of practicing physicians. | http://www.onemedicine.com |
| *Nature's Herbs*<br>Jim Duke, editor<br>A detailed description of herbs commonly used in the United States. | http://www.herbalvillage.com/<br>article1.html |
| *Queensland Herb Society Newsletter*<br>Australian newsletter containing links to herb resources. | http://www.powerup.com.au/~sage/ |
| *Townsend Letter for Doctors and Patients*<br>Jonathan Collin, M.D., publisher<br>Scientific and anecdotal information from researchers, health practitioners, and patients. | http://www.tldp.com/ |

paperbacks geared toward consumers, and newsletters written for clinicians, administrators, or consumers. An extensive range of online newsletters is available, geared to every conceivable audience, and most all the various types of Web sites listed develop and tailor content for their readers continuously (Table 7-3).

## CONCLUSION

Internet information on CAM (Tables 7-4 and 7-5) is proliferating at an unprecedented rate, and substantial shifts are occurring in the scientific base and research in-

*Text continued on p. 115*

**TABLE 7-4** Evidence-Based Resources in Complementary and Alternative Medicine

| DATABASE | ACCESS | URL |
|---|---|---|
| **Bandolier**<br>*Complementary Medicine Summaries*<br>Bandolier is a print and Internet journal about health care, using evidence-based medicine techniques to provide advice about particular treatments or diseases for health care professionals and consumers. The content is tertiary publishing, distilling the information from (secondary) reviews of (primary) trials and making it comprehensible. Bandolier contains more than 75 summaries on the effectiveness of complementary therapies. | Free | http://www.jr2.ox.ac.uk/ bandolier/booth/booths/ altmed.html |
| **CAM on PubMed**<br>CAM on PubMed was developed jointly by the National Library of Medicine (NLM) and NCCAM to help persons search easily for journal articles related to a variety of CAM therapies, approaches, and systems. CAM on PubMed contains 220,000 citations, has links to full text, and allows searchers to limit retrievals by publication type. To search, go to the subsets menu and select "Complementary Medicine." | Free | http://www.ncbi.nlm.nih. gov/entrez/query.fcgi? CMD=Limits&DB= PubMed |
| **CISCOM**<br>The Centralized Information Service for Complementary Medicine (CISCOM) of the Research Council for Complementary Medicine, United Kingdom, contains 4000 randomized trials and more than 60,000 citations and abstracts covering and arranged by the major complementary therapies including acupuncture, aromatherapy, healing, hypnotherapy, chiropractic, homeopathy, and manipulation. | Fee to access | http://www.rccm.org.uk/ cisc.htm |
| **Cochrane Complementary Medicine Field Registry**<br>*Complementary Medicine Field*<br>To meet the growing need for evidence-based complementary medicine, the Complementary Medicine Field promotes and facilitates the production and collection of systematic reviews in complementary medicine and continually maintains and updates a registry of randomized controlled trials. The registry is located at the University of Maryland Complementary Medicine Program. | Free | http://www.compmed. umm.edu/cochrane/ index.html |

*Continued*

**TABLE 7-4** Evidence-Based Resources in Complementary and Alternative Medicine—cont'd

| DATABASE | ACCESS | URL |
|---|---|---|
| **Cochrane Library**<br>*Cochrane Collaboration*<br>The Cochrane Library is an electronic publication produced by the Cochrane Collaboration to supply high-quality evidence to inform persons providing and receiving care and those responsible for research, teaching, funding, and administration. The database is published quarterly on CD-ROM and the Internet and is distributed by subscription. The database contains more than 5600 reports of randomized controlled trials and more than 83 systematic reviews in complementary medicine. | Fee to access | http://www.cochrane library.com/clibhome/ clib.htm |
| **HerbMed**<br>HerbMed is an herbal database that provides hyperlinked access to the scientific data underlying the use of herbs for health and is an evidence-based information resource for professionals, researchers, and the general public. HerbMed contains 125 evidence-based reviews of herbal therapies. | Free | http://www.herbmed.org/ |
| **Ovid Best Evidence Collection**<br>More than 90 journals on internal medicine and other specialties such as family practice, pediatrics, obstetrics, psychiatry, gynecology, and surgery are scanned, and only those articles that meet strict selection criteria for study design are selected for review. The articles are summarized in a structured abstract, with expert commentary. The collection can be searched separately but also is available as a limit (EBM reviews) from MEDLINE. The collection contains more than 1500 full-text reports on complementary medicine. | Fee to access | http://www.ovid.com |
| **POEMs: Patient Oriented Evidence That Matters**<br>*Journal of Family Practice*<br>POEMs features reviews of more than 90 journals and identifies the eight articles most important for primary care clinicians to read. POEMs contains coverage of complementary therapies. | Free | http://www.infopoems.com/ |

| TABLE 7-4 Evidence-Based Resources in Complementary and Alternative Medicine—cont'd | | |
|---|---|---|
| **DATABASE** | **ACCESS** | **URL** |
| **SUMSearch**<br>*University of Texas Health Science Center*<br>SUMSearch is a unique method of searching for medical evidence by using the Internet. SUMSearch combines metasearching and contingency searching to automate searching for medical evidence. SUMSearch covers complementary therapies. | Free | http://www.uthscsa.edu/ |
| **TRIP Database**<br>*National Health Service, United Kingdom*<br>The TRIP Database searches 58 sites of high-quality medical information and gives direct, hyperlinked access to the largest collection of evidence-based material on the Web, as well as articles from premier online journals such as the *British Medical Journal, Journal of the American Medical Association,* and *New England Journal of Medicine.* The database contains evidence-based information on complementary and alternative therapies. | Free | http://www.tripdatabase.com/ |
| **University of Maryland Complementary Medicine Program Databases**<br>This program facilitates systematic literature reviews and evaluation. Other databases include the Arthritis and Complementary and Alternative Medicine Database (ARCAM) and the Complementary and Alternative Medicine and Pain Database (CAMPAIN). | Free | http://www.compmed.umm.edu/ |

## TABLE 7-5 Databases for Research in Complementary and Alternative Medicine

| DATABASE | ACCESS | URL |
|---|---|---|
| **ACUBASE**<br>Published by the Bibliothéque Universitatire de Médicine de Nîmes, this database contains more than 11,000 French and English references and full-text articles dedicated specifically to the discipline of acupuncture. The database also includes conference proceedings. | Fee to access | http://www.trigram.com/default.htm |
| **ACULARS**<br>Contains about 40,000 citations from journals published in more than 10 languages in the fields of acupuncture, moxibustion, acupuncture anesthesia, and meridians. | Fee to access | wulc@sun.ihep.ac.cn (e-mail) |
| **AGRICultural OnLine Access (AGRICOLA)**<br>This bibliographic database of citations to the agricultural literature was created by the National Agricultural Library and its cooperators and includes citations for herbs and medicinal plants and includes references from HerbalGram of the Herb Research Foundation. | Free | http://www.nal.usda.gov/ag98/ |
| **Allied and Complementary Medicine (AMED)**<br>AMED is a unique database produced by the Health Care Information Service of the British Library and includes resources for complementary medicine, palliative care, and several professions allied with medicine. AMED is available in a variety of formats, from print to online. | Fee to access | http://www.bl.uk/ |
| **AltHealthWatch**<br>*EBSCO Information Services*<br>This is a Web-based, full-text database of periodicals, peer-reviewed journals, academic and professional publications, magazines, consumer newsletters and newspapers, research reports, and associations. | Fee to access | http://www.epnet.com/eptech/ |
| **CAM on PubMed**<br>*National Center for Complementary and Alternative Medicine*<br>The bibliographic citations are obtained from the NLM MEDLINE database that uses a feature to locate citations with predetermined CAM search criteria. | Free | http://www.nlm.nih.gov/nccam/camonpubmed.htm |

**TABLE 7-5** Databases for Research in Complementary and Alternative Medicine—cont'd

| DATABASE | ACCESS | URL |
|---|---|---|
| CAMline<br>CAMline is an evidence-based Web site on CAM for health care professionals and the public and represents a successful collaboration of conventional and CAM organizations, interests, and expertise. | Free | http://www.ars-grin.gov/duke/index.html |
| ClinicalTrials.gov<br>This site provides current information on disease treatment at particular institutions or by a disease, drug, modality, therapy, or procedure. The site contains complementary and alternative medicine therapies (search by words: "alternative" [medicine or therapy] or "complementary" [medicine or therapy], by particular modality [acupuncture], or by a particular substance [ginko or shark cartilage]). | Free | http://clinicaltrials.gov/ |
| Cumulative Index to Nursing and Allied Health (CINAHL)<br>CINAHL indexes alternative medicine journals. | Fee to access | http://www.cinahl.com/ |
| Datadiwan<br>Datadiwan provides access to information on holistic medicine and frontier sciences. Second, Datadiwan is a scientific discussion forum in which interested parties can discuss scientific topics with other like-minded persons around the world. Third, Datadiwan is a network that links research institutions and organizations worldwide. Most of the literature is in German. | Free | http://www.datadiwan.de/index_e.htm |
| Dr. Duke's Phytochemical and Ethnobotanical Databases<br>*Agricultural Research Service, U.S. Department of Agriculture (ARS, USDA)*<br>The ARS, USDA, databases can be searched by chemical, specific activity, or ethnobotanical usage. | Free | http://www.ars-grin.gov/duke/index/html |
| EMBASE<br>This international database contains citations covering the biomedical, pharmacological, and drug literature. | Fee to access | http://www.embase.com/ |

*Continued*

| TABLE 7-5 Databases for Research in Complementary and Alternative Medicine—cont'd | | |
|---|---|---|
| **DATABASE** | **ACCESS** | **URL** |
| **EthnobotDB (Plant Uses Worldwide)** James A. Duke and Stephen M. Beckstrom-Sternberg, of the National Germplasm Resources Laboratory (NGRL), ARS, USDA, built this database, which contains 80,000 records of plant uses. | Free | http://www.ars-grin.gov/duke/index/html |
| **HerbMed** This herbal database provides hyperlinked access to the scientific data underlying the use of herbs for health and is an evidence-based information resource for professionals, researchers, and general public. The database is a project of the Alternative Medicine Foundation. | Free | http://www.herbmed.org/ |
| **Hom-Inform Database** This database of indexed literature references in homeopathy is produced by the British Homeopathic Library at Glasgow Homeopathic Hospital and is searchable online. | Free | http://hominform.soutron.com/ |
| **International Bibliographic Information on Dietary Supplements (IBIDS)** This database is produced by the Office of Dietary Supplements, NIH, along with the Food and Nutrition Information Center, National Agricultural Library, USDA. IBIDS contains bibliographic records, including abstracts published in international scientific journals on the topic of dietary supplements, including vitamins, minerals, and herbal and botanical supplements. The general public, scientists, researchers, and others can search the database using keywords to obtain the citations of research journal articles. | Free | http://ods.od.nih.gov/databases/ibids.html |
| **Manual, Alternative and Natural Therapy (MANTIS) Database (formerly CHIROLARS)** Coverage for health care disciplines not represented significantly in the major biomedical databases. References are from more than 1000 journals, with preference given to peer-reviewed journals. MANTIS includes health promotion and prevention, acupuncture, allopathic medicine, alternative medicine, chiropractic, herbal medicine, homeopathy, naturopathy, osteopathic medicine, physical therapy, and Chinese medicine. | Fee to access | http://www.healthindex.com |

| TABLE 7-5 Databases for Research in Complementary and Alternative Medicine—cont'd | | |
|---|---|---|
| DATABASE | ACCESS | URL |
| Medicinal Plants of Native America Database (MPNADB) This database "contains 17,634 items representing the medicinal uses of 2,147 species from 760 genera and 142 families by 123 different native American groups—was built over a period of about 10 years with support from the National Endowment for the Humanities, the National Science Foundation, and the University of Michigan-Dearborn." | Free | http://www.umd.umich.edu/cgi-bin/herb |
| MEDLINE/PubMed The best interface is PubMed from the NLM, Bethesda, Maryland. The MEDLINE database supports the teachings and research of the current medical system in the United States. The database contains 11 million citations and includes the complementary medicine subset CAM on PubMed. | Free | http://www.ncbi.nlm.nih.gov/entrez/ http://www.nlm.nih.gov/nccam/camonpubmed.html |
| MICROMEDEX Complementary & Alternative Medicine (CAM) Series The Complementary & Alternative Medicine Series from MICROMEDEX is a comprehensive, clinically focused reference tool based on a thorough compilation of scientific literature. Monographs in the series present data on administration, dosing, warnings, precautions, contraindications, and interactions. | Fee to access | http://www.micromedex.com/products/healthcare/cam/si-8753.pdf |
| MICROMEDEX Herbal & Alternative Remedies *American Academy of Family Physicians, familydoctor.org* This database of alternative medicines has an alphabetically arranged index and allows searches by name. Information is provided by AltCareDex and is produced by MICROMEDEX Thomson Healthcare products. | Fee to access | http://www.familydoctor.org/cgi-bin/altcaredex_search |
| Native American Ethnobotany Database Dan Moerman, professor of anthropology at the University of Michigan-Dearborn, describes the database as "foods, drugs, dyes, fibers and other uses of plants (a total of over 47,000 items). This represents uses by 291 Native American groups of 3,895 species from 243 different plant families." | Free | http://www.umd.umich.edu/cgi-bin/herb |

*Continued*

**TABLE 7-5** Databases for Research in Complementary and Alternative Medicine—cont'd

| DATABASE | ACCESS | URL |
|---|---|---|
| **Natural Medical Protocols for Doctors** <br> This Web-accessible fee-based service "includes current research data and treatment protocols for most common medical conditions and cross-linked reference material about vitamins, minerals, herbs, homeopathy and other supplements and therapies." | Fee to access | http://www.natmedpro.com/ |
| **Natural Medicines Comprehensive Database** <br> *Pharmacist's Letter/Prescriber's Letter* <br> This database provides clinical data on the natural medicines, herbal medicines, and dietary supplements used in the Western world and is compiled by pharmacists and physicians. | Fee to access | http://www. naturaldatabase.com/ |
| **Natural Products ALERT (NAPRALERT)** <br> *STN International* <br> This database contains bibliographic and factual data on natural products, including information on the pharmacology, biological activity, taxonomic distribution, ethnomedicine, and chemistry of plant, microbial, and animal (including marine) extracts. | Fee to access | http://info.cas.org/ ONLINE/DBSS/ napralertss.html |
| **Nutritionals Adverse Event Monitoring System** <br> *U.S. FDA, Center for Food Safety & Applied Nutrition, Office of Special Nutritionals* <br> This database of adverse effects is compiled from the use of special nutritional products—dietary supplements, infant formulas, and medical foods—as reported by health professionals and consumers. | Free | http://www.cfsan.fda.gov/ |
| **Patent Database** <br> *U.S. Patent and Trademark Office* <br> This tool locates registered patents in complementary and alternative medicine. | Free | http://www.uspto.gov/ patft/index.html |
| **PhytoNet** <br> *Centre for Complementary Health Studies, University of Exeter* <br> PhytoNet is a "resource for those involved in the development, manufacture, regulation and surveillance of phytomedicines and herbal drugs" and contains information from the European Scientific Co-operative on Phytotherapy (ESCOP), forms to submit adverse effects of herbal medicines, and European standards for safe use of phytomedicines. | Free | http://www.escop.com/ phytonet.htm |

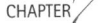

**TABLE 7-5** Databases for Research in Complementary and Alternative Medicine—cont'd

| DATABASE | ACCESS | URL |
|---|---|---|
| **Phytotherapies.org Monograph Database**<br>This database is a free service to individuals registering with the site and is "sponsored by Herbworx Corporation, an Australian company dedicated to ensuring that practitioners are supplied not only with high quality herbal medicine, but also clinically relevant, scientifically validated technical information, and Phytomedicine manufacturer quality herbal extracts for practitioners." Even though the service is commercial, the herbal monograph database contains indications, actions, constituents, studies, and articles. | Free | http://www.phytotherapies.org/ |
| **Poisonous Plant Database**<br>*U.S. FDA, Center for Food Safety & Applied Nutrition, Office of Plant and Dairy Foods and Beverages*<br>The Poisonous Plant Database is a set of working files of scientific information about animal and human toxicology of vascular plants of the world. | Free | http://vm.cfsan.fda.gov/~djw/readme.html |
| **PsychInfo**<br>*American Psychological Association*<br>PsychoInfo is a source for mind-body and other complementary and alternative therapies used in mental disorders, stress reduction, or psychological and behavioral processes and neuroimmunology. | Fee to access | http://www.apa.org/psycinfo/ |

frastructure. The Internet offers access to CAM information provided by many different organizations and agencies. This information overload can make searching the Internet for CAM information a frustrating and time-consuming process. Additionally, the disaggregation of CAM information on the Internet can lead to potential knowledge gaps between health professionals and patient-consumers. In the next chapter we cover CAM Internet-based information initiatives and the impact of the Internet on health consumers. In many cases, information that is geared toward health professionals is also of value to health consumers and patients. Consequently, some overlap occurs with the information provided in Chapter 7. There is also overlap in this chapter with material presented in Chapter 3 on doing a general search for CAM information.

## References

1. Berman BM and others: Primary care physicians and complementary-alternative medicine: training, attitudes, and practice patterns, *J Am Board Fam Pract* 11(4):272-281, 1998.
2. Astin JA: Why patients use alternative medicine: results of a national study, *JAMA* 279(19):1548-1553, 1998.
3. Ernest E, Cassileth BR: The prevalence of complementary/alternative medicine in cancer: a systematic review, *Cancer* 83(4):777-782, 1998.
4. Berman BM: The Cochrane Collaboration and evidence-based complementary medicine, *J Altern Complement Med* 3(2):191-194, 1997.
5. Ezzo J and others: Complementary medicine and the Cochrane Collaboration, *JAMA* 280(18):1628-1630, 1998.
6. Chalmers I, Dickersin K, Chalmers TC: Getting to grips with Archie Cochrane's agenda, *BMJ* 305(6857):786-788, 1992.
7. Dickersin K, Manheimer E: The Cochrane Collaboration: evaluation of health care and services using systematic reviews of the results of randomized controlled trials, *Clin Obstet Gynecol* 41(2):315-331, 1998.

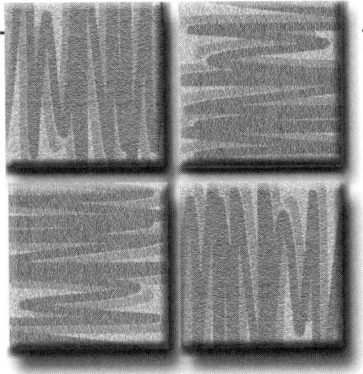

# Complementary and Alternative Medicine and Consumer Health Information on the Internet

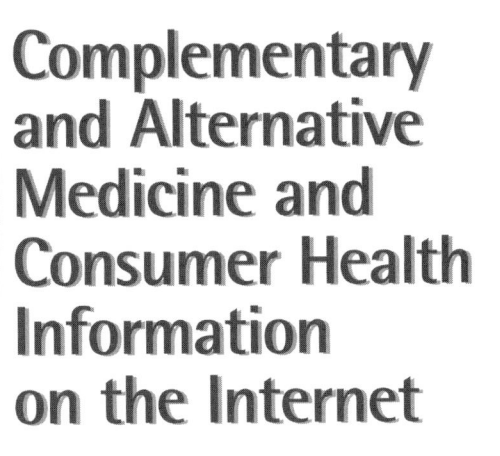

**Chapter Highlights**
Introduction
Health Consumer Use of the Internet
Types of Users and Medical Conditions
Quality and Safety Issues
Resources for Consumers and Patients

## INTRODUCTION

Health care providers increasingly are treating patients who are bringing Internet printouts to consultations. These printouts often include information on CAM products and practices. Current estimates on the frequency of this phenomenon vary from 58%[1] to more than 70%.[2] Although the impact of this access to health information on the practitioner-patient relationship has been debated,[3] the Internet increasingly is playing a role in medical decision making and is empowering patients to become more involved in health care decision making.

## HEALTH CONSUMER USE OF THE INTERNET

Much of the limited evidence as to who the consumers of Internet health information are and what they are looking for comes from market research surveys and Web use statistics, both quantifying the numbers of users and types of information accessed. Women are more likely than men to seek health care information online, and the highest proportion of use is among those between 30 and 64 years old.[4] Use of the Internet for health information declines with age.[5,6] Despite the much-discussed digital divide between the higher-income, more-educated individuals and the lower-income, less-educated individuals, little evidence indicates that differences in seeking of health information vary by income group once Internet access has been achieved.[7]

A 1999 Harris Poll of 2000 adults in the United States found that mental health issues dominated the most popular online health topics, with depression, bipolar disorder, and anxiety problems accounting for 42% of Web use to find health information.[8] Most users research specific health issues that currently are affecting a friend, relative, or themselves, frequently in connection with a visit to their doctor. Few use health sites to communicate with health services, purchase pharmaceuticals, or participate in health-related chat-room discussions.[4] However, most users in the United States report a desire for more online interaction with their doctors, including e-mail consultations and reminders.[9]

Users report valuing the convenience, anonymity, and volume of online information.[9]

##  TYPES OF USERS AND MEDICAL CONDITIONS

The California Healthcare Foundation has categorized three types of users[10]:
1. The well
2. The newly diagnosed
3. The chronically ill and their caregivers

The well group carries out episodic searching for information relating to short-term medical conditions, pregnancy, and prevention issues. The newly diagnosed group carries out intensive searching for specific information, valuing the ease of access and broad range of information. The chronically ill and their caregivers carry out regular searching for information related to new treatments, nutrition advice, and alternative therapies.

In addition, the latter two groups value and use online communities and chat rooms. Several studies have shown the importance of the World Wide Web in providing social support, particularly to individuals with chronic health problems such as diabetes[11] or individuals with HIV.[12]

### Use of Complementary and Alternative Health Information

Limited data exist on users of CAM information on the Internet. The data that do exist suggest that those seeking CAM information on the Internet are primarily those who suffer from chronic illness and that they are seeking general information on CAM and nutritional advice. As trends in user involvement, consumer empowerment, and wide dissemination of information on CAM continue, understanding and addressing the needs and desires of those who are accessing CAM information on the Internet will become increasingly more important. The resources discussed in the following sections can help patients and consumers who are considering CAM treatments.

### Government Resources

#### National Center for Complementary and Alternative Medicine

NCCAM is dedicated to exploring complementary and alternative healing practices in the context of rigorous science, training CAM researchers, and disseminating author-

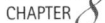

itative information to health care consumers and patients. The Web site is **<http://nccam.nih.gov/>**.

### National Center for Complementary and Alternative Medicine Public Information Clearinghouse

As one of its mandates from Congress, NCCAM is charged with "the dissemination of health information in respect to identifying, investigating, and validating complementary and alternative treatment, diagnostic and prevention modalities, disciplines, and systems" (Public Law 105-277). The NCCAM Public Information Clearinghouse serves this mission and is the point of contact for the public for scientifically based information on CAM and for information about NCCAM. One may contact the center by mail, telephone, or e-mail or may visit the Web site.

National Center for Complementary and Alternative Medicine
P.O. Box 7923
Gaithersburg, MD 20898
Telephone: 1-888-644-6226; outside the United States: (301) 519-3153
Fax: 1-866-464-3616 (toll-free)
TTY: 1-866-464-3615 (toll-free)
E-mail: info@nccam.nih.gov
http://nccam.nih.gov/health/clearinghouse/index.htm

NCCAM also provides additional resources for the public:

**Acupuncture**
http://nccam.nih.gov/health/acupuncture/index.htm
**Cancell/Entelev**
http://cis.nci.nih.gov/fact/9_13.htm
**Coenzyme Q$_{10}$**
http://cis.nci.nih.gov/fact/9_16.htm
**Complementary and alternative medicine therapies**
http://nccam.nih.gov/health/advice/index.htm
**Frequently asked questions about CAM and NCCAM**
http://nccam.nih.gov/htdig/search.html
**General information about NCCAM**
http://nccam.nih.gov/htdig/search.html
**Hepatitis** C
http://nccam.nih.gov/health/hepatitisc/index.htm
**Laetrile/amygdalin**
http://cis.nci.nih.gov/fact/9_3.htm
**NCCAM Newsletter**
http://nccam.nih.gov/news/newsletter/fall2001/1.htm
**NCCAM Public Information Clearinghouse**
http://nccam.nih.gov/health/clearinghouse/index.htm
**NCCAM research grants: Information for researchers**
http://nccam.nih.gov/htdig/search.html
**St. John's wort**
http://nccam.nih.gov/health/stjohnswort/index.htm

### CAM on PubMed

CAM on PubMed, which has more than 220,000 citations, is accessed through the PubMed database, which also includes MEDLINE. Sponsored by NCCAM, PubMed can be accessed at <http://www.nlm.nih.gov/nccam/camonpubmed.html>.

### Combined Health Information Database

The federally supported CHID is another service in which NCCAM participates, which includes a variety of materials not available in other government databases. CHID aggregates health information for the public on numerous topical areas related to health and disease at <http://chid.nih.gov/>.

### National Cancer Institute

NCI has funded a number of CAM clinical trials, many with NCCAM, including evaluation of the value of vitamins and minerals in cancer prevention and treatment, Gonzales nutritional therapy, angiogenesis effects of shark and bovine cartilage, the effects of carotenoid nutrients on human papilloma viral lesions, the effect of natural inhibitors of carcinogenesis, and other types of natural products research. The Web site is <http://www.nci.nih.gov/>.

*Office of Cancer and Complementary and Alternative Medicine.* The Office of Cancer Complementary and Alternative Medicine (OCCAM) was established in October 1998 to coordinate and enhance the activities of NCI concerning CAM. The

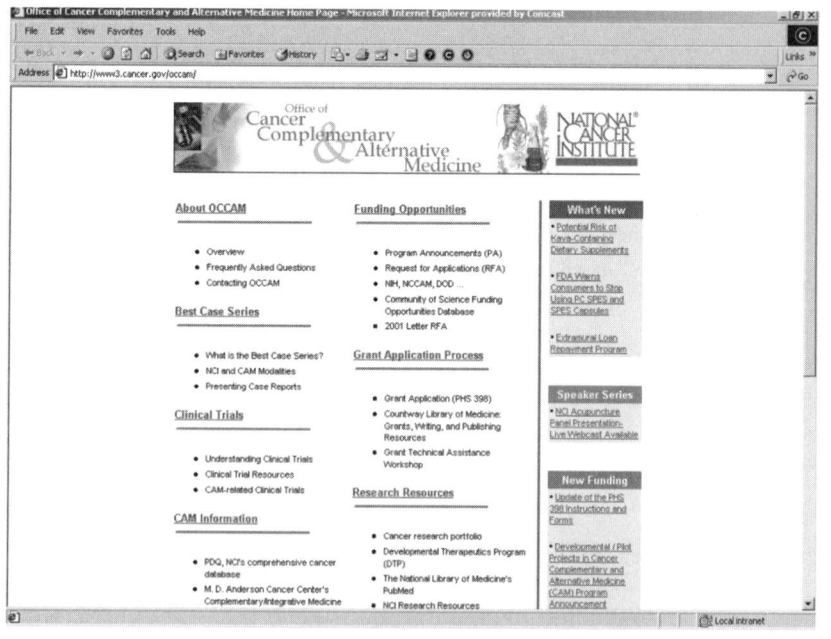

FIG. 8-1  ■  Home page of the Office of Cancer and Complementary and Alternative Medicine.

goal of OCCAM is to increase the amount of high-quality cancer research and information about the use of complementary and alternative modalities. The Web site is <http://www3.cancer.gov/occam/> (Fig. 8-1).

*Cancer Trials Database.* NCI also provides a database on cancer trials at <http://www.nci.nih.gov/clinical_trials/>.

---

## ■ QUALITY AND SAFETY ISSUES

### Food and Drug Administration

The FDA regulates dietary supplements under a set of regulations different from those covering conventional foods and drug products (prescription and over-the-counter). Under DSHEA the dietary supplement manufacturer is responsible for ensuring that a dietary supplement is safe before marketing it. The FDA is responsible for taking action against any unsafe dietary supplement product after it reaches the market. Generally, manufacturers do not need to register with the FDA or get FDA approval before producing or selling dietary supplements. Manufacturers must make sure that product label information is truthful and not misleading. The postmarketing responsibilities of the FDA include monitoring safety (for example, voluntary dietary supplement adverse event reporting) and product information such as labeling, claims, package inserts, and accompanying literature. The FDA Web site is **<http://www. fda.gov/>** (Fig. 8-2).

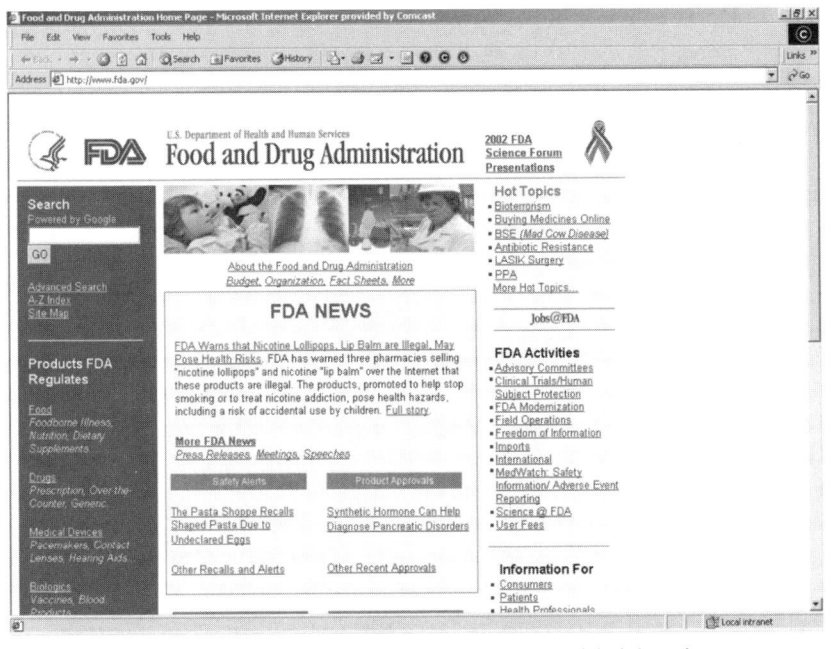

FIG. 8-2  ■  Home page of the Food and Drug Administration.

The FDA provides a food safety site at <http://www.cfsan.fda.gov/> and dietary supplements/food labeling electronic newsletter at <http://www.cfsan.fda.gov/~dms/fda-dsfl.html>.

## Centers for Disease Control and Prevention

In the area of CAM the CDC has taken a role in monitoring herbal supplements and also has analyzed data on nutritional supplements. Although the CDC Web site does not post material dedicated specifically to alternative medicine, a subject search yielded 40 documents, primarily reports in portable document format. All entries are ranked by relevance to the topic. Of the first 20, 19 were published within the past 15 months. The CDC site also provides excellent up-to-date information regarding infectious diseases, outbreaks, and epidemiology at <http://www.cdc.gov/> (Fig. 8-3).

## Federal Trade Commission

The FTC protects consumers by pursuing organizations that fraudulently market products and services on the Web. Recent enforcement actions have been taken and are currently under way. The FTC Web site is <http://www.ftc.gov/opa/2001/06/cureall.htm>.

## The World Health Organization

WHO provides an excellent report entitled *World Health Organization Report: The Strategy for Traditional Medicine for 2002-2005*.

## Canadian Natural Health Products Directorate

The Canadian Natural Health Products Directorate has the authority to approve natural health products for the Canadian market, ensuring Canadian consumers safe natural health products. The Web site is <http://www.hc-sc.gc.ca/hpb/onhp/welcome_e.html>.

## Health Protection Branch, Canada

The Health Protection Branch of Canada regulates and controls supplies such as medical devices, product safety, and drugs. The Web site is <http://www.hc-sc.gc.ca/hpb/>.

# RESOURCES FOR CONSUMERS AND PATIENTS

## National Center for Complementary and Alternative Medicine Clinical Trials

NCCAM funds and monitors more CAM research than any other institution in the United States. The level of appropriation for NCCAM has been increased twice, to a budget of $113 million for the year 2003. Because of the funding and partnerships with other sections of the NIH, NCCAM has achieved aggregate funding totaling roughly $200 million for 2002. Table 7-1 provides a list of clinical trials for which subjects currently are being recruited.

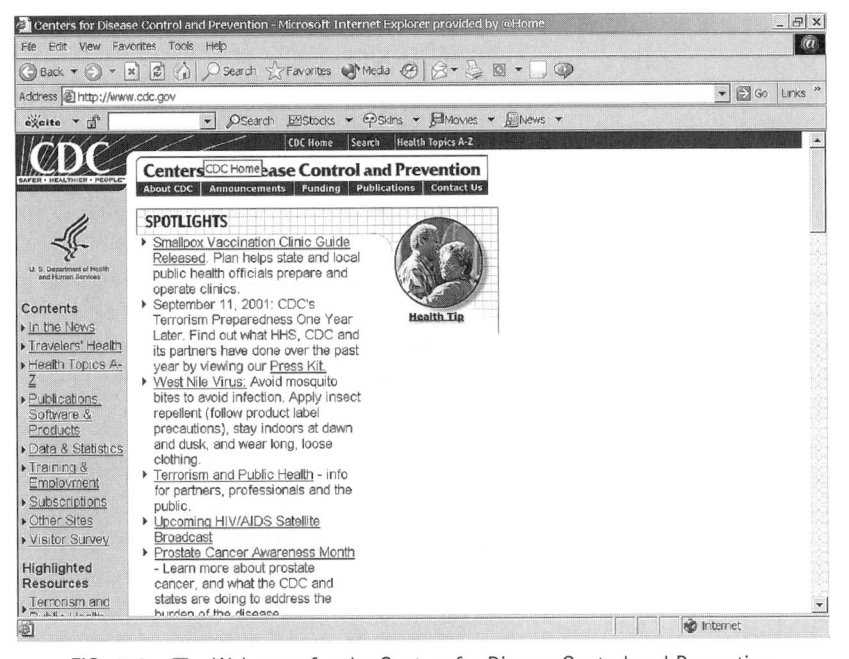

FIG. 8-3  ■  Web page for the Centers for Disease Control and Prevention.

## ClinicalTrials.gov

ClinicalTrials.gov provides a complete listing of all CAM trials sponsored by the NIH. For a complete listing of clinical studies in CAM, one should search under the keyword *"alternative medicine."* As of April 2002, 147 clinical trials were listed at <http://www.clinicaltrials.gov/>.

In addition to funding individual clinical trials, NCCAM has funded or provided additional funding for 15 research centers in the United States. Each program concentrates on prevention and treatment of at least one major disease condition or on the health issue of a particular population. These centers in turn have the ability to fund pilot studies known as development-of-feasibility projects. Given the focus of each of these centers, they are in a position to conduct, assess, and stimulate research within their respective areas of study. Quite a few research organizations now are focused on complementary medicine; most often these are academic medical schools that are involved in performing research and teaching medical students. A number of them also have developed integrative clinics where patients are treated. Some institutions, such as the University of Maryland, include a focus on informatics.

## MEDLINEplus

Designed for health professionals and consumers, MEDLINEplus has extensive information from the NIH and other trusted sources on about 500 diseases and conditions including CAM treatments. MEDLINEplus also provides lists of hospitals and physicians, a medical encyclopedia and dictionaries, health information in Spanish, extensive information on prescription and nonprescription drugs, health information from the media, and links to thousands of clinical trials. The Web site is <http://www.nlm.nih. gov/medlineplus/alternativemedicine.html>.

## Healthfinder

Healthfinder is a massive directory that provides links to Web sites and is essentially a searchable health portal linked to preselected quality government and private health-related sites, including those on complementary therapies. Healthfinder can be searched by broad topic, by diagnosis, and by therapy and is linked primarily to Web resources and organizations. A search of the keyword *"alternative medicine"* produced a list of 149 resources on the Web and 66 organizations. The Web site is <http://www.healthfinder.gov/>.

## White House Commission on Complementary and Alternative Medicine Policy

President Clinton formed WHCCAMP to make recommendations on public policy and legislation pertaining to complementary and alternative medicine. The Web site contains the full White House commission report and transcripts of town hall meetings at <http://www.whccamp.hhs.gov/>.

## Information Sources from Canada and the United Kingdom

### Cochrane Consumer Network

Table 8-1 lists summaries of Cochrane Systematic Reviews for consumers.

### Bandolier

Bandolier strives to gather the best evidence available about CAM for patients, consumers, and professionals and to update this information as better evidence becomes available. The Web site is **<http://www.jr2.ox.ac.uk/Bandolier/booth/booths/altmed.html>**.

### Organising Medical Networked Information

OMNI is a gateway to evaluated, quality Internet resources in health and medicine aimed at students, researchers, academics, and practitioners in the health and medical sciences. The Web site is **<http://omni.ac.uk/>**.

## Complementary and Alternative Medicine Directories

Heathwell
Comprehensive information regarding alternative health and integrative medicine
http://www.healthwell.com
**McMaster University Alternative Medicine Resources**
A comprehensive Canadian directory of Web sites on the Internet
http://www-hsl.mcmaster.ca./tomflem/altmed.html

| | TABLE 8-1 Summaries of Cochrane Systematic Reviews for Consumers | |
|---|---|---|
| THERAPY | SUMMARY OR TITLE | URL |
| Acupuncture | Acupuncture does not appear to help smokers who are trying to quit | http://www.cochraneconsumer.com/Content.ASP?ID=CO0000000009 |
| Acupuncture | Acupuncture might be able to provide short-term relief from tennis elbow, but more research is needed | http://www.cochraneconsumer.com/Content.ASP?ID=CO0000001269 |
| Acupuncture | Acupuncture seems to be able to help relieve headaches and migraine, but more reliable research is needed | http://www.cochraneconsumer.com/Content.ASP?ID=CO0000000924 |
| Acupuncture | Not enough evidence exists about acupuncture for asthma, and more research is needed | http://www.cochraneconsumer.com/Content.ASP?ID=CO0000000007 |
| Alexander technique | No evidence that the Alexander technique can relieve asthma symptoms or reduce the need for medication, and more research is required | http://www.cochraneconsumer.com/Content.ASP?ID=CO0000000013 |
| Herbal therapies | Evening primrose oil may be acceptable to people with schizophrenia and may have a moderately positive effect | http://www.cochraneconsumer.com/Content.ASP?ID=CO0000000684 |
| Herbal therapies | Title: "St John's wort for depression" | http://www.cochraneconsumer.com/Content.ASP?ID=CO0000000797 |
| Herbal therapies | The herbal remedy feverfew might be able to prevent migraines, but more reliable research is needed | http://www.cochraneconsumer.com/Content.ASP?ID=CO0000000322 |
| Herbal therapies | Title: "Herbal therapy for treating rheumatoid arthritis" | http://www.cochraneconsumer.com/Content.ASP?ID=CO0000000959 |
| Herbal therapies | Vitamin $B_1$ and magnesium may help reduce the pain of dysmenorrhoea | http://www.cochraneconsumer.com/Content.ASP?ID=CO0000001126 |
| Herbal therapies | Title: "Chinese medicinal herbs for chronic hepatitis B" | http://www.cochraneconsumer.com/Content.ASP?ID=CO0000000939 |
| Herbal therapies | Not enough evidence on whether methenamine (hexamine) salts can prevent urinary tract infection, but they have few adverse effects and might help | http://www.cochraneconsumer.com/Content.ASP?ID=CO0000001313 |

*Continued*

**TABLE 8-1** Summaries of Cochrane Systematic Reviews for Consumers—cont'd

| THERAPY | SUMMARY OR TITLE | URL |
|---------|------------------|-----|
| Herbal therapies | Herbal medicines used in combination with interferons for people with hepatitis C have not been shown to be effective | http://www.cochraneconsumer.com/Content.ASP?ID=CO0000001230 |
| Herbal therapies | Extracts of the traditional South Pacific plant remedy and recreational drug, kava, may provide effective relief from anxiety | http://www.cochraneconsumer.com/Content.ASP?ID=CO0000001223 |
| Herbal therapies | Extracts from the African prune tree (*Pygeum africanum*) may be able to help relieve urinary symptoms caused by enlarged prostate | http://www.cochraneconsumer.com/Content.ASP?ID=CO0000001329 |
| Herbal therapies | Title: "Herbal therapy for treating osteoarthritis" | http://www.cochraneconsumer.com/Content.ASP?ID=CO0000000958 |
| Herbal therapies | There is weak evidence that some Chinese medicine may help hepatitis B in symptom-free people carrying the virus, but more research is needed | http://www.cochraneconsumer.com/Content.ASP?ID=CO0000001018 |
| Homeopathy | Homeopathic *Oscillococcinum* does not prevent influenza, but probably shortens the length of the illness | http://www.cochraneconsumer.com/Content.ASP?ID=CO0000000368 |
| Homeopathy | Not enough evidence from trials to determine whether or not homeopathy can help improve asthma | http://www.cochraneconsumer.com/Content.ASP?ID=CO0000000367 |
| Homeopathy | There is not enough evidence to show the effect of homeopathy for inducing labour | http://www.cochraneconsumer.com/Content.ASP?ID=CO0000001212 |
| Prayer | Title: "Intercessory prayer for the alleviation of ill health" | http://www.cochraneconsumer.com/Content.ASP?ID=CO0000000412 |
| Tai Chi | Interventions to prevent falls in elderly people can be effective | http://www.cochraneconsumer.com/Content.ASP?ID=CO0000000432 |
| Yoga | No reliable evidence to support the use of yoga as a treatment for control of epilepsy | http://www.cochraneconsumer.com/Content.ASP?ID=CO0000000914 |
| Yoga | Not enough evidence about the use of breathing exercises (including yoga and the Buteyko method) by people with asthma | http://www.cochraneconsumer.com/Content.ASP?ID=CO0000000126 |

**New York Online Access to Health (NOAH)**
Complementary and alternative medicine
http://www.noah-health.org/english/alternative/alternative.html
**Rosenthal Center**
A comprehensive and authoritative listing from Columbia University in New York of
    complementary and alternative medicine resources
http://cpmcnet.columbia.edu/dept/rosenthal/
**University of Pittsburgh**
Alternative medicine home page
http://www.pitt.edu/~cbw/altm.html
**Yahoo Alternative Medicine**
A listing of more than 500 CAM sites
http://dir.yahoo.com/Health/Alternative_Medicine/

## Web Sites

**Ask Dr. Weil**
DrWeil.com is a leading provider of online information and products for optimum
    health and wellness.
http://www.drweil.com/app/cda/drw_cda.php
**InteliHealth**
A comprehensive CAM site with a broad range of timely information
http://www.intelihealth.com/IH/ihtIH/WSIHW000/8513/8513.html?k=navx408x8513
**MedWebPlus: Alternative Medicine**
Extensive directory of CAM sites organized using the same alternative medicine med-
    ical subject headings used by the National Library of Medicine.
http://www.medwebplus.com/subject/Alternative_Medicine.html
**WebMD/Medscape**
WebMD/Medscape is a comprehensive site offering Internet-based medical informa-
    tion for consumers and professionals. The site includes extensive content on alter-
    native and complementary medicine resources for patients. Registration is required.
http://www.medscape.com/
**WholeHealthMD**
WholeHealthMD.com is a partnership between leading companies in health care:
    American WholeHealth and Rebus.
http://www.wholehealthmd.com/

## Topical Sites and News

The value of news for researchers is its topical nature, reporting on what is being published in the scientific and medical literature. These sites also may report on use, new
developments, and trends in the field. Staying abreast of complementary medicine is
important and requires scanning topical sources in the media, including newspapers,
magazines, newsletters, and the Web, for new therapies and new research. Just because a controlled clinical trial has not been performed does not represent proof that
a therapy does, or does not, work. Epidemiological data and trends are other types of

information available from news sources. In the context of how one gathers and synthesizes information, topical content has relevance.

**ABC News.com: Health & Living News Index**
http://www.abcnews.com/sections/Living/

**TABLE 8-2** Selected Associations for Complementary and Alternative Medicine

| ASSOCIATION | MODALITY | COUNTRY | URL |
|---|---|---|---|
| American Academy of Medical Acupuncture | Acupuncture | United States | http://www.medicalacupuncture.org/ |
| American Association of Naturopathic Physicians | Naturopathy | United States | http://www.naturopathic.org/ |
| American Chiropractic Association | Chiropractic | United States | http://www.amerchiro.org/ |
| American Herbal Products Association | Herbal medicine | United States | http://www.ahpa.org/ |
| American Herbalists Guild | Herbal medicine | United States | http://www.healthy.net/herbalists/ |
| American Holistic Medical Association | Holistic medicine | United States | http://holisticmedicine.org/ |
| American Massage Therapy Association | Massage | United States | http://www.amtamassage.org/ |
| Association of Physical and Natural Therapists | Herbal and manual therapies | United Kingdom | http://www.apnt.org.uk/ |
| British Chiropractic Association | Chiropractic | United Kingdom | http://www.chiropractic-uk.co.uk/ |
| British Herbal Medicine Association | Herbal medicine | United Kingdom | http://info.ex.ac.uk/phytonet/bhma.html |
| British Homeopathic Association | Homeopathy | United Kingdom | http://www.trusthomeopathy.org/trust/tru_over.html |
| British Medical Acupuncture Society | Acupuncture | United Kingdom | http://www.medical-acupuncture.co.uk/ |
| Canadian Chiropractic Association | Chiropractic | Canada | http://www.ccachiro.org/ |
| Complementary Medicine Association | Complementary medicine | United Kingdom | http://www.the-cma.org.uk/ |
| National Center for Homeopathy | Homeopathy | United States | http://www.healthy.net/nch/ |
| Touch for Health Association | Therapeutic touch | United States | http://www.tfhka.org/ |

**Alternative Health News Online**
http://www.altmedicine.com/FrameSet.asp
**CNN daily updates on health topics**
http://www.medscape.com/Home/Topics/multispecialty/multispecialty.html
**Health Watch**
http://www.hwatch.org/index.shtml
**HealthWell Natural News**
http://www.healthwell.com/news/index.cfm
**Medscape Medical Research News**
http://www.medscape.com/medscapetodayhome
**Natural Health Line**
http://www.naturalhealthvillage.com/
*New York Times* **Daily Health News: Your Health Daily**
http://yourhealthdaily.com/
**Reuters Health Information Services, Inc.**
http://www.reutershealth.com/
**Science Daily News**
http://www.sciencedaily.com/index.htm
*USA Today* **Health**
http://www.usatoday.com/life/health/health.htm

## Newsletters

The Internet meets an important need by providing and disseminating information on alternative therapies. Links between the publishing industry and the Internet reflect the breadth of the technology transfer that is taking place, through books and content that include medical textbooks, texts used in the training of CAM professionals, quality CAM journals, full-text journal articles available online, quality trade paperbacks geared toward consumers, and newsletters written for clinicians, administrators, or consumers. An extensive range of online newsletters is available, geared to every conceivable audience, and most of the Web sites listed develop and tailor content for their readers continuously. (See Table 7-3 for a list of newsletters on CAM.)

Table 8-2 lists selected associations that provide information on CAM.

## References

1. Impact of the Internet on primary care staff in Glasgow, *J Med Internet Res* 1(2):E7, 1999.
2. Hjortdahl P, Nylenna M, Aasland OG: Internet and the physician-patient relationship: from "thank you" to "why"? *Tidsskr Nor Laegeforen* 119(29):4339-4341, 1999.
3. Gerber BS, Eiser AR: The patient-physician relationship in the Internet age: future prospects and the research agenda, *J Med Internet Res* 3(2):E15, 2001.
4. Fox SR: *The Pew Internet and American Life Project: the online health care revolution: how the Web helps Americans take better care of themselves,* November 26, 2000, The Pew Charitable Trust.
5. Smith-Barbaro PA and others: Factors associated with intended use of a Web site among family practice patients, *J Med Internet Res* 3(2):E17, 2001.

6. Licciardone JC, Smith-Barbaro PA, Coleridge ST: Use of the Internet as a resource for consumer health information: results of the Second Osteopathic Survey of Health Care in America (OSTEOSURV-II), *J Med Internet Res* 3(4):E31, 2001.

7. Brodie M and others: Health information, the Internet, and the digital divide, *Health Aff* (Millwood) 19(6):255-265, 2000.

8. Taylor H: *The Harris Poll #47: explosive growth of "cyberchondriacs" continues*, 1999.

9. *Cybercitizen Health 2001*, Cyber Dialogue, 2001, *http://www.cyberdialogue.com.*

10. Cain MM MR, Sarasohn-Kahn J, Wayne JC: *Health e-people: the online consumer experience*, Oakland, CA, 2000, California Healthcare Foundation and the Institute for the Future.

11. Zrebiec JF, Jacobson AM: What attracts patients with diabetes to an Internet support group? A 21-month longitudinal Website study, *Diabet Med* 18(2):154-158, 2001.

12. Reeves PM: Coping in cyberspace: the impact of Internet use on the ability of HIV-positive individuals to deal with their illness, *J Health Commun* 5(suppl):47-59, 2000.

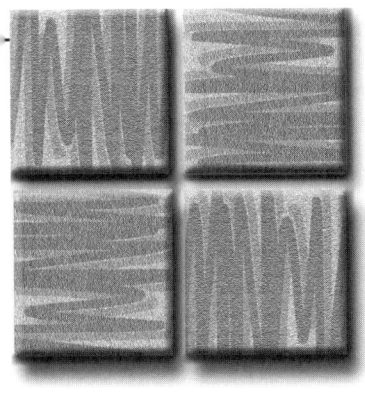

# Legal, Ethical, and Privacy Issues

**Chapter Highlights**
Introduction
Complementary and Alternative Medicine and
  Informed Consent
Physician-Patient and Provider-Patient Relationships
Quality Information and Ethics of Medical and Health
  Care Web Sites
Privacy and Security
Licensing and Record Keeping
Conclusion

## INTRODUCTION

The popularity of CAM among patient-consumers seeking health care poses serious challenges for health care professionals. The issues and obstacles involving integrative health initiatives in CAM arise from the fact that interest and use of CAM therapies have developed faster than the guidelines and principles needed for practitioners to incorporate CAM practices into the current framework of conventional medical practice. This disparity is further compounded by Internet-enabled communications between physicians and patients regarding CAM therapies.

## COMPLEMENTARY AND ALTERNATIVE MEDICINE AND INFORMED CONSENT

An important factor regarding physician-patient communications on CAM is informed consent. Informed consent in CAM, as in conventional medicine, should include adequate information about the potential risks and benefits of CAM therapies. Failure to provide information regarding the safety and efficacy of CAM therapies can result in dissatisfied patients and increase the potential for malpractice claims.[1] Informed consent is also an important factor for physicians making decisions regarding referrals to CAM practitioners.

The information needed by the patient to ensure informed decision making and consent includes the following:

- The probability of benefit
- The potential for harm or risk associated with the procedure
- The alternative options available and their associated risks and benefits

Requirements for informed consent dictate that patients be made aware of benefits and risks of the therapy in question. Physicians and health care professionals need to have access to the best available information on the safety and efficacy of CAM therapies and should discuss with patients the potential risk and benefits of CAM therapies. Doing so can increase patient satisfaction and reduce the risks of malpractice lawsuits. A number of initiatives such as the Cochrane Collaboration Complementary Medicine Field provide access to up-to-date evidence-based summaries of the latest research in CAM, including systematic reviews and consumer-oriented summaries of systematic reviews in CAM. For medical professionals the Cochrane Library is perhaps the most comprehensive source for high-quality systematic reviews of CAM. In addition, numerous commercial, academic, and organizational databases are available online and on CD-ROM that provide valid up-to-date information on the safety and quality of CAM therapies and products, including herbals and dietary supplements. Also up-to-date society information can be obtained from Web sites such as the FTC and FDA and from commercial sites such as consumerlab.com.

 ## PHYSICIAN–PATIENT AND PROVIDER–PATIENT RELATIONSHIPS

Patients who are looking for treatment options are going online and becoming savvier about their choices in health care; they also desire more online contact with their physicians. As more online communications occur, ethical considerations are being raised as to how online communications are to be defined regarding the physician-patient relationship. Do the physician and patient have to meet in person or just converse to have a relationship? Does a physician consultant to a Web site have an ethical obligation to visitors? Do certain types of services carry more liability than others? Current case law has not yet defined where and at what point the physician-patient relationship begins when the only contact between the two is online. However, several initiatives have begun to try to tackle the difficulties associated with online communications between physicians and patients. The eRisk Working Group in Healthcare,[2] in cooperation with more than a dozen U.S. medical societies and 30 malpractice carriers representing greater than 70% of the insured physicians in the United States, has developed guidelines to help guide physician-patient communications on the Internet.

## QUALITY INFORMATION AND ETHICS OF MEDICAL AND HEALTH CARE WEB SITES

Inevitably, health care professionals are asked to recommend useful Web sites in CAM. As mentioned in previous chapters, great concern exists regarding the accuracy and quality of many CAM Web sites, particularly sites with a primary purpose of e-commerce. Ensuring quality online content in CAM is and will continue to be a persistent challenge. Physicians and patients must be aware of what information is available, the source of the information, and the intended audience. Additionally, physicians should be able to discuss quality initiatives and the recent development of guidelines that allow patient-consumers to rate health information on the Internet as physicians seek to guide patients in making their own decisions about the validity of CAM Web sites (see Table 4-1). Even though many health Web sites now provide seals of approval and awards, recent data suggests that three out of four Internet users seeking health information feel that a doctor's recommendation would make them more likely to trust a health Web site.[3] By providing this information, physicians can influence positively patient selection of online material. Unfortunately, less than 5% of patients report getting Web site information from their physicians. This trend likely will change as the popularity of physician practice Web sites continues to increase, as evidenced in a recent corporate survey in which pediatric practices with Web sites increased from 24% to 46% from August 1999 to October 2000.[2]

##  PRIVACY AND SECURITY

Perhaps the most critical issue regarding online communications is the right of privacy. In this age of ever-expanding access to information, ensuring the privacy of online interactions is critical. This is understandably one of the most sensitive issues among those seeking health information on the Internet.[3] Such concern needs to extend beyond physician communications and include the need for secure Web sites that prevent personal medical information, including patterns of use and interests, from being sold, purchased, or inadvertently placed in the hands of marketers, employers, and insurers.[4]

The U.S. government currently is taking steps to protect online privacy and to ensure the confidentiality of medical records. The Health Insurance Portability and Accountability Act (HIPAA) of 1996, which will be implemented in 2003, will begin to govern the privacy of medical records and protect digital health and health-related information. The law will require providers, claims clearinghouses, and health plans to comply with more stringent regulation of patient data and to implement administrative and technical steps to protect the confidentiality of electronic health records[5] (Fig. 9-1).

Medical data and anti-paparazzi laws included in HIPAA may yet be extended to allow victims to sue for damages that occur from an online information broker obtaining personal medical information. In addition, future cyberstalking laws[6] could be expanded to include obtaining medical information via the Internet. If adapted, both laws could go a long way toward preventing private medical information from getting into the wrong hands. However, even if more U.S. regulations are enacted, they are only enforceable in the United States. Ultimately, online activities and behaviors may require international regulation to standardize medical and health care Internet conduct.

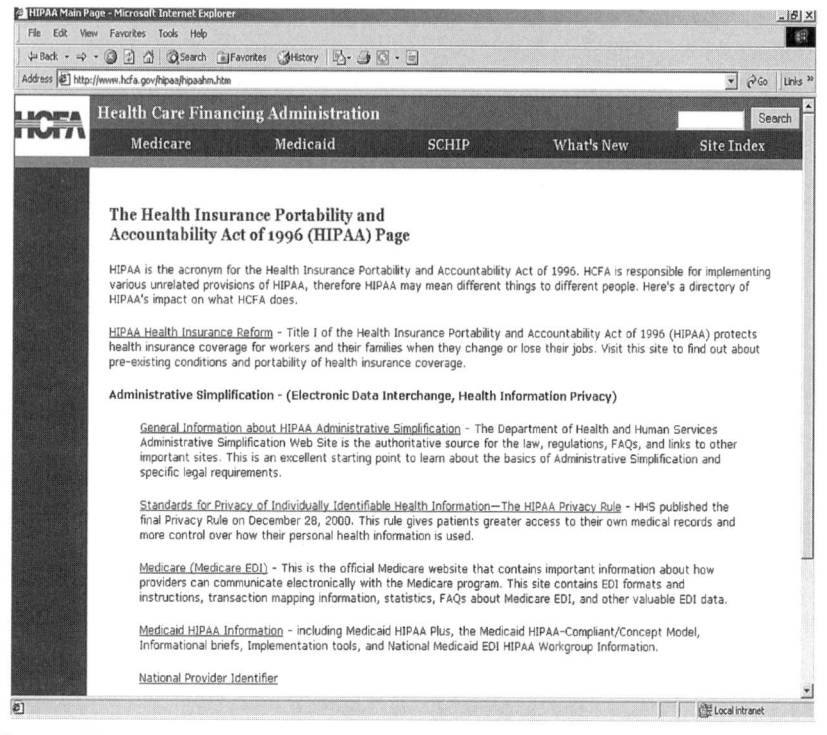

**FIG. 9-1** ■ Web page for the Health Insurance Portability and Accountability Act of 1996.

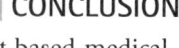 ## LICENSING AND RECORD KEEPING

Another issue regarding online communications is that of licensing. In conventional medicine, conventional physicians and CAM practitioners are licensed to practice within a given state. With e-mail and the capability to converse freely across state and national borders, patients and consumers now have greater access to physicians via physician Web sites. Thus the issue of licensing will need to be addressed as more health care providers and patients interact online. Currently, California is the only state with an in-state telemedicine license. In addition, when online communications occur, the policies, procedures, and technology must be in place to ensure that important health information is captured and retained as part of the patient record.[7]

## CONCLUSION

Internet-based medical, health, and CAM information will play an increasingly important role in health care as greater numbers of patient-consumers turn to the Internet for health and medical information. As these developments and technical innovations transform health care, they will introduce many new ethical challenges

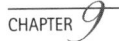

for practitioners, patients, and consumers as medical information merges with the Internet.

## References

1. Informed consent in complementary and alternative medicine, *Arch Intern Med* 161(19):2288-2292, 2001.
2. Medem Inc: Risk for providers: understanding and mitigating provider risk associated with online patient interaction, *http://www.medem.com/erisk* (accessed March 2001).
3. Fox SR: *The Pew Internet and American Life Project: the online health care revolution: how the Web helps Americans take better care of themselves,* November 26, 2000, The Pew Charitable Trust.
4. Winker MA and others: Guidelines for medical and health information sites on the Internet: principles governing AMA web sites, *JAMA* 283(12):1600-1606, 2000.
5. Russo H: HIPAA: Creating privacy protection that works, *Caring* 20(5):12-16, 2001.
6. California Department of Consumer Affairs, Legislative Digest SB 1796: *Stalking: cyberstalking,* Civil Code Section 1708.7 and Penal Code Section 422, 1998, pp 646.9, 653.
7. Medem Inc: eRisk guidelines: for physician-patient online communications, *http://www.medem.com/erisk* (accessed March 2001).

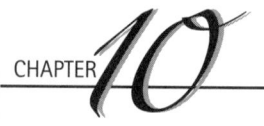

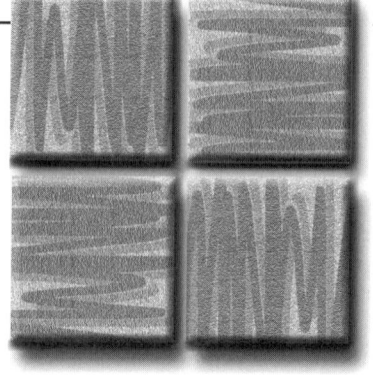

# The Future

**Chapter Highlights**
Introduction
Assumptions
Challenges
Vision for the Future

## INTRODUCTION

The Internet now serves as a vital link between the tremendous volume of health information generated by research and the means for the rapid and widespread dissemination and exchange of that information.[1] Use of the Internet in health care is commonplace. Publications from the *New York Times* to the *Journal of the American Medical Association* have featured stories on how consumers are finding medical information on the Internet and are taking a more active role in their care. Health care professionals also are using the Internet increasingly to keep up in their fields, to communicate with patients, and to consult with one another.

Consumers' interest in and use of CAM therapies are inseparable. Data from Eisenberg and others[2] found that 42% of the U.S. population had used CAM in the previous year. CAM is popular on the Internet as well. A search using Google and the keyterm *"alternative medicine"* yields more than 500,000 hits (Google search, November 2001, <**www.google.com**>). To date, however, little comprehensive data is available on Internet use by those who use CAM.

## 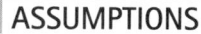ASSUMPTIONS

To help evaluate the scenario of the future, the authors have made the following assumptions:

1. Health professionals and consumers increasingly will use computers and the Internet as means of collecting, communicating, and transacting health information.
2. Independent of advances in the scientific knowledge of CAM therapies, improvements in computer technology and high-speed access to the Internet by health consumers and patients will continue.
3. Decision support systems providing timely information on the safety, efficacy, and quality of CAM interventions and products at the point of care will be developed.

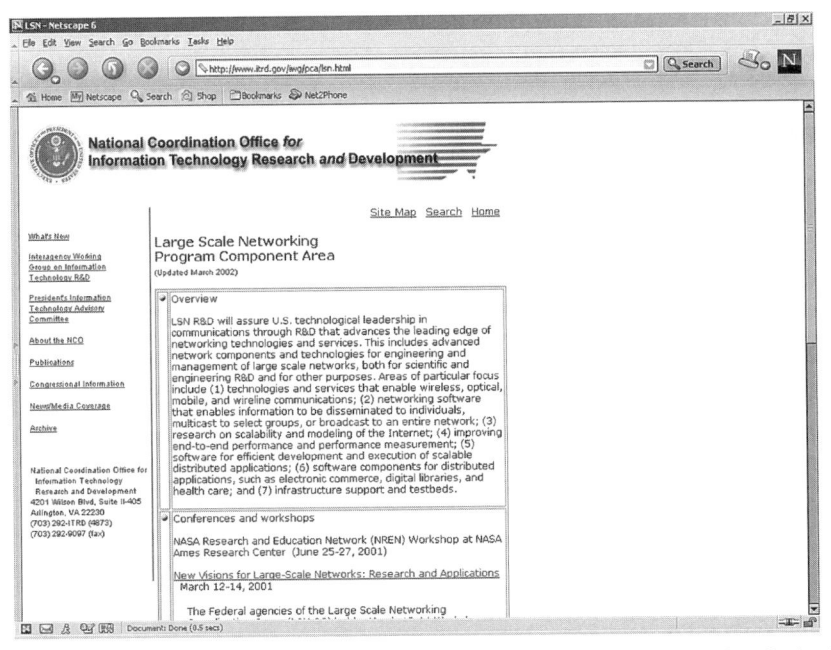

FIG. 10-1  ■  Home page for the National Coordination Office for Information Technology Research and Development.

4.  Challenges will exist in standardizing CAM terminologies, organizing and collecting large-scale databases, and in determining levels of evidence for incorporation into best practices (Fig. 10-1).

## CHALLENGES

The growth of interest and research in CAM and the ability to access and transfer CAM information via the Internet will present many challenges in the future.

### Lack of Professional Standards in Complementary and Alternative Medicine Terminology and Definition

One challenge is that no widely accepted, controlled vocabulary is in use from which to build expert systems. In biomedical databases such as MEDLINE and EMBASE, indexing of CAM literature is incomplete, making locating relevant research difficult. In addition, much of the literature on CAM is scattered among many online and print sources, and these are inconsistent in how they define CAM and index CAM literature. For example, Chinese movement therapies such as *qi gong* and *tai chi* are considered complementary therapies by the Cochrane Collaboration Complementary Medicine Field but are not accessed by a MEDLINE search of the MeSH term "*alternative medicine.*" Similarly, herbal remedies may be described by MEDLINE as plant extracts rather than by any alternative medicine term.[3]

## Quality of Health Information on the Internet

As greater numbers of consumers access the Internet for health information, many unresolved issues remain regarding the quality, relevance, and organization of the health information available. The Internet provides many benefits, but its unique qualities, including its broad reach and relative anonymity, have given rise to Web sites peddling fraudulent and even dangerous CAM drugs and devices to health care consumers. For example, the FDA has warned consumers to stop taking the dietary supplement/herbal product PC-SPES because it contains undeclared prescription drug ingredients that are potentially deadly if not used with medical supervision. PC-SPES products were sold as immune enhancers and for prostate health. The company producing these products issued a recall and is now no longer in business.

## Limits of Scientific Knowledge in Complementary and Alternative Medicine

Many questions still remain to be answered regarding the effectiveness and safety of complementary therapies, and much remains to be accomplished in the rigorous collection, evaluation, and dissemination of high-quality information in CAM. Recent surveys continue to show growth in the interest and use of CAM therapies worldwide by health care professionals who increasingly are being called on to make thoughtful, informed, evidence-based recommendations regarding CAM.[2,4]

## Collaboration

As research funding in CAM continues to increase worldwide and as greater numbers of studies are published annually, the need for synthesized evidence in CAM will continue to grow. This evidence, in the form of systematic literature reviews, increasingly is becoming recognized as the best means of synthesizing medical information.[5] Therefore as the research base in CAM matures, a tremendous need will arise for a coordinated international effort among researchers, health care professionals, policy makers, and consumers to provide up-to-date, high-quality systematic reviews on CAM treatments.

An existing model of this type of international collaboration is the Cochrane Collaboration. With more than 6000 members worldwide, the Cochrane Collaboration aims to provide reliable, high-quality, evidence-based information by preparing, maintaining, and promoting the conduct and accessibility of systematic reviews of all available evidence regarding the benefits and risks of health care.[6] Currently, the Cochrane Library alone has more than 1000 published systematic reviews and several hundred protocols in progress. The library is fast approaching a doubling in size with the release of every issue. Within the Cochrane Library, there exists systematic reviews of CAM treatments, and new reviews are underway.

## ■ VISION FOR THE FUTURE

High-speed, next-generation Internet (NGI) combined with advances in computing technologies will allow for a proliferation of tools and applications that have the potential to transform health care and the conduct of biomedical research. In CAM, these applications will foster the continuing analysis, integration, and dissemination of results of basic science and clinical research.

Advances in information technology (including networking, databases, and computer methods for collecting, analyzing, and visualizing data from individuals and populations) will offer unprecedented opportunities to enhance the quality of research and patient care. In addition, these technologies will enhance the efficiency with which new knowledge can be generated, analyzed, and integrated into medicine.

For patients and consumers, new technologies have the potential to allow for the rapid dissemination of high-quality educational and research information, thus allowing for more effective monitoring and follow-up by providing feedback loops for connecting providers, patient-consumers, and researchers (Fig. 10-2). Table 10-1 outlines how these technologies can be used to generate information that serves health care professionals, patients, and consumers.

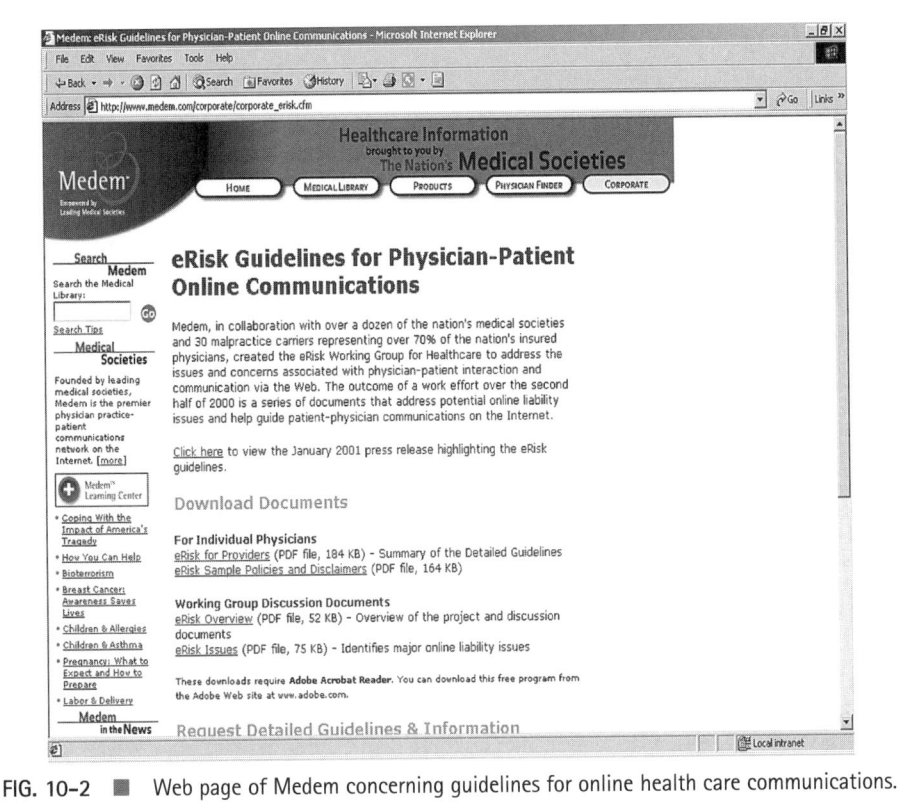

FIG. 10–2 ■ Web page of Medem concerning guidelines for online health care communications.

**TABLE 10-1 Technology and Uses for Generating Information in Complementary and Alternative Medicine**

| APPLICATION/ TOOLS | NEEDS OF MEDICAL PROFESSIONALS: MEDICAL INFORMATICS | INFORMATION NEEDS OF HEALTH CONSUMERS |
|---|---|---|
| Ongoing clinical research | Databases of randomized controlled trials for professionals<br>Databases of synthesized medical evidence<br>Systematic reviews<br>Meta-analyses | Databases of trials for consumers and consumer-based summaries of the best medical evidence (Cochrane Consumer Network) |
| Decision support | Clinical systems for professionals and expert systems for management of patients who are using CAM or who want to include CAM in treatment | Decision-making tools for patients, such as for checking symptoms, assessing risk, and provision of self-care options |
| Medical documentation | Health record systems and electronic patient records | Patient-accessible health records (Internet health records), patient-held health records (smart cards), electronic patient health diaries, and patients' personal Web pages |
| Information retrieval | Bibliographic and factual databases (e.g., CAM on PubMed), specialized databases, and portals to medical knowledge | Consumer-oriented bibliographic and factual databases (MEDLINEplus, databases of randomized controlled trials)<br>Health portal Web sites and evaluated directories of information |
| Education and training | Web-based digital libraries containing information on medical education, continuing medical education (CME) opportunities, fellowships, and training opportunites | Health education and promotion of EBM and CAM |
| Drug information | Pharmacy systems and national and international drug interaction surveillance with herbal and nutritional products | Patient-accessible systems to check interactions between drugs and between drugs, herbals, nutritional supplements, and foods |

## References

1. What's up in medical informatics? *CMAJ* 157(12):1718-1719, 1997 (miscellaneous).
2. Eisenberg DM and others: Trends in alternative medicine use in the United States, 1990-1997: results of a follow-up national survey, *JAMA* 280(18):1569-1575, 1998.
3. Ezzo J and others: Complementary medicine and the Cochrane Collaboration, *JAMA* 280(18):1628-1630, 1998.
4. Eisenberg DM: Advising patients who seek alternative medical therapies, *Ann Intern Med* 127(1):61-69, 1997.
5. Smith R, Chalmers I: Britain's gift: a "Medline" of synthesised evidence, *BMJ* 323(7327): 1437-1438, 2001.
6. Chalmers I, Dickersin K, Chalmers TC: Getting to grips with Archie Cochrane's agenda, *BMJ* 305(6857):786-788, 1992.

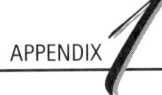
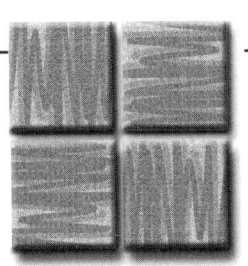

# The Cochrane Collaboration Complementary Medicine Field

*"It is surely a great criticism of our profession that we have not organized a critical summary, by specialty or subspecialty, adapted periodically, of all relevant randomized controlled trials."*

ARCHIE COCHRANE, 1906-1988

## MISSION

The Cochrane Collaboration is an international organization that brings together health care providers, consumers, and scientists who volunteer to compile up-to-date systematic reviews of evidence regarding the benefits and risks of health care. The Cochrane Collaboration publishes these reviews quarterly in the Cochrane Library.

## HISTORY

The Cochrane Collaboration takes its name from physician and humanitarian Archie Cochrane. Dr. Cochrane believed in and strongly advocated producing systematic reviews of the medical literature as a way of creating "evidence-based medicine." A systematic review assembles all the results of clinical research studies in a given health topic and uses explicit methods to minimize bias (systematic errors) and random error (simple mistakes) in determining the safety and effectiveness of an intervention. Dr. Cochrane felt that for a clinician to keep up with the volumes of information being generated was not humanly possible and that properly conducted reviews would provide an objective summary of large amounts of data. His vision was the creation of an organization whose sole purpose was to conduct systematic reviews in every aspect of medicine.

The importance of systematic reviews of scientific evidence, rather than traditions, common practices, or case histories, is well illustrated in the following true story. In 1972 the first study was published examining whether a course of an inexpensive drug (a corticosteroid) given to women expected to give birth prematurely could help reduce complications in the infant. Additional trials were done over the next 15 years, appearing periodically in the medical literature. However, it took a systematic review summarizing all the trials to establish beyond a doubt that giving this drug reduced the odds of babies dying from complications by 30% to 50%. Because the systematic review had not been published until 1989, most obstetricians did not know that the treatment was so effective, even though evidence had existed since 1972. As a result, tens of thousands of premature babies may have suffered and died unnecessarily.

With the formation of the Cochrane Collaboration in 1993, Archie Cochrane's vision became a reality.

## COCHRANE LIBRARY

The main product of the Cochrane Collaboration, the Cochrane Library, contains the full text of more than 1200 completed, up-to-date Cochrane reviews (Table AI-1) and more than 900 protocols of reviews (Table AI-2) in progress. Several hundred newly completed reviews and protocols are added each year. This effort results from more than 6000 persons in 60 counties working collectively and systematically to collect, evaluate, and disseminate systematic reviews in all aspects of health care. The library is published quarterly on CD-ROM and the Internet and is distributed to subscribers.

In addition, the Cochrane Collaboration maintains the Cochrane Controlled Trials Registry, which contains more than 300,000 controlled clinical trials that are published electronically in the Cochrane Library and via the Internet <http://www.update-software.com/>. This electronic format allows reviewers to update or modify Cochrane reviews in response to new evidence or comments and criticisms from readers. In responding to the needs of consumers for high-quality health care information, the Cochrane Consumer Network <http://www.cochraneconsumer.com/> was established within the Cochrane Collaboration in 2001 to help promote the interests of users of health care and to provide and disseminate rigorous and relevant consumer-based summaries of Cochrane reviews.

## COCHRANE COLLABORATION STRUCTURE

Three types of groups work within the collaboration: collaborative review groups (CRGs), centers, and fields. CRGs are arranged by disease specialty. Approximately 51 CRGs now represent disease areas such as diabetes, depression, upper respiratory tract infections, and musculoskeletal disorders. The review groups are responsible for doing systematic reviews related to their disease specialty. Cochrane centers (presently 15) exist to support the CRGs, whereas fields (19) represent the interests of a specific group of patients (such as elderly or teens) or a specific type of treatment (such as physical therapy). Fields, such as the Complementary Medicine Field, work in collaboration with the CRGs to produce systematic reviews.

*Text continued on p. 157*

## TABLE AI-1 Cochrane Reviews in Complementary Medicine

| AUTHORS | REVIEW TITLE | YEAR-ISSUE OR AMENDMENT | COCHRANE COLLABORATIVE REVIEW GROUP |
|---|---|---|---|
| 1. Casimiro L, Brosseau L, Milne S, Robinson V, Wells G, Tugwell P | Acupuncture and electroacupuncture for the treatment of RA [rheumatoid arthritis] | 2002, *Issue* 3 | Musculoskeletal |
| 2. Linde K, Jobst K, Panton J | Acupuncture for chronic asthma | 1996, *Issue* 3 | Airways |
| 3. Melchart D, Linde K, Fischer P, Berman B, White A, Vickers A, Allais G | Acupuncture for idiopathic headache | 2001, *Issue* 1 | Chronic Pain, Palliative Care, and Supportive Care |
| 4. Smith CA, Crowther CA | Acupuncture for induction of labour | 2001, *Issue* 1 | Pregnancy and Childbirth |
| 5. Green S, Buchbinder R, Hall S, Barnsley L, Forbes A, Smidt N, Assendelft W | Acupuncture for lateral elbow pain in adults | 1999, *Issue* 1 | Musculoskeletal |
| 6. Tulder MW, van Cherkin DC, Berman B, Lao L, Koes BW | Acupuncture for low back pain | 1999, *Issue* 1 | Back |
| 7. White AR, Rampes H, Ernst E | Acupuncture for smoking cessation | 1997, *Issue* 1 | Tobacco and Addictions |
| 8. Dennis J | Alexander technique for chronic asthma | 2000, *Issue* 2 | Airways |
| 9. Evans JR, Henshaw K | Antioxidant vitamin and mineral supplements for preventing age-related macular degeneration | 1999, *Issue* 4 | Eyes and Vision |
| 10. Evans JR | Antioxidant vitamin and mineral supplements for age-related macular degeneration | 1998, *Issue* 1 | Eyes and Vision |
| 11. Nixon S, O'Brien K, Glazier RH, Wilkins AL | Aerobic exercise interventions for people with HIV/AIDS | 2001, *Issue* 1 | HIV/AIDS |

*Continued*

# TABLE AI-1 Cochrane Reviews in Complementary Medicine—cont'd

| AUTHORS | REVIEW TITLE | YEAR-ISSUE OR AMENDMENT | COCHRANE COLLABORATIVE REVIEW GROUP |
| --- | --- | --- | --- |
| 12. McIntosh HM, Olliaro P | Artemisinin derivative for treating uncomplicated malaria | 1998, *Issue* 2 | Infectious Disease |
| 13. Pittler MH, Thompson Coon J, Ernst E | Artichoke leaf extract for treating hypercholesterolaemia | 2002, *Issue* 3 | Heart Group |
| 14. McIntosh HM, Olliaro P | Artemisinin derivatives for treating severe malaria | 1998, *Issue* 3 | Infectious Disease |
| 15. Verhagen AP, De Vet HCW, de Bie RA, Kessels AGH, Boers M, Knipschild PG | Balneotherapy for rheumatoid arthritis and osteoarthritis | 1999, *Issue* 3 | Musculoskeletal |
| 16. Brazzelli M, Griffiths P | Behavioural and cognitive interventions for faecal incontinence in children | 2001, *Issue* 1 | Incontinence |
| 17. Norton C, Hosker G, Brazzelli M | Biofeedback and sphincter exercises for treatment of faecal incontinence in adults | 2000, *Issue* 2 | Incontinence |
| 18. Wilt T, Ishani A, MacDonald R, Stark G, Mulrow C, Lau J | Beta-sitosterols for benign prostatic hyperplasia | 2000, *Issue* 2 | Prostatic Diseases/Urological Cancer |
| 19. Karjalainen K, Malmivaara A, van Tulder M, Roine R, Jauhiainen M, Hurri H, Koes B | Biopsychosocial rehabilitation for upper limb repetitive strain injuries | 2000, *Issue* 3 | Musculoskeletal Injuries |
| 20. Holloway E, Ram FSF | Breathing exercises for asthma | 1998, *Issue* 4 | Airways |
| 21. Hoare C, Leonard T, Williams HC | Chinese herbal medicine for atopic eczema | 2000, *Issue* 2 | Skin |

| | | | | |
|---|---|---|---|---|
| 22. | Wilt T, MacDonald R, Ishani A, Rutks I, Stark G | Cernilton for benign prostatic hyperplasia | 1998, *Issue 2* | Prostatic Diseases/Urological Cancer |
| 23. | Liu JP, McIntosh H, Lin H | Chinese medicinal herbs for chronic hepatitis B | 2001, *Issue 1* | Hepato-Biliary |
| 24. | Price JR, Couper J | Cognitive behavior therapy for chronic fatigue syndrome in adults | 1998, *Issue 3* | Depression, Anxiety, and Neurosis |
| 25. | Jones C, Cormac I, Mota J, Campbell C | Cognitive behavior therapy for schizophrenia | 1999, *Issue 1* | Depression, Anxiety, and Neurosis |
| 26. | Jepson RG, Mihaljevic L, Craig J | Cranberries for the prevention of urinary tract infections | 1998, *Issue 4* | Renal |
| 27. | Brosseau L, Casimiro L, Milne S, Robinson V, Shea B, Tugwell P, Wells G | Deep transverse friction massage for treating tendinitis | 2002, *Issue 1* | Musculoskeletal |
| 28. | Jepson RG, Mihaljevic L, Craig J | Cranberries for the treatment of urinary tract infections | 1998, *Issue 4* | Renal |
| 29. | Woods RK, Thien FCK, Abramson MJ | Dietary marine fatty acids (fish oil) for asthma | 2000, *Issue 3* | Airways |
| 30. | Van den Ende CHM, Vliet Vlieland TPM, Munneke M, Hazes JMW | Dynamic exercise therapy for rheumatoid arthritis | 2000, *Issue 3* | Musculoskeletal |
| 31. | Flemming K, Cullum N | Electromagnetic therapy for treatment of pressure sores | 2000, *Issue 3* | Wounds |
| 32. | Melchart D, Linde K, Fischer P, Kaesmayr J | Echinacea for the prevention and treatment of the common cold | 1999, *Issue 1* | Acute Respiratory Infections |
| 33. | Busch A, Schachter CL, Peloso PM, Bombardier C | Exercise for treating fibromyalgia syndrome | 2002, *Issue 3* | Musculoskeletal |

*Continued*

| AUTHORS | REVIEW TITLE | YEAR-ISSUE OR AMENDMENT | COCHRANE COLLABORATIVE REVIEW GROUP |
| --- | --- | --- | --- |
| 34. Flemming K, Cullum N | Electromagnetic therapy for treatment of pressure sores | 2001, *Issue* 1 | Wounds |
| 35. Hulme J, Robinson V, DeBie R, Wells G, Judd M, Tugwell P | Electromagnetic fields for the treatment of osteoarthritis | 2001, *Issue* 1 | Musculoskeletal |
| 36. Flemming K, Cullum N | Electromagnetic therapy for the treatment of venous leg ulcers | 2001, *Issue* 1 | Wounds |
| 37. Pittler MH, Vogler BK, Ernst E | Feverfew for preventing migraine | 2000, *Issue* 3 | Pain, Palliative Care, and Supportive Care |
| 38. Farmer A, Montori V, Dinneen S, Clar C | Fish oil in people with type II diabetes | 2001, *Issue* 3 | Metabolic and Endocrine Disorders |
| 39. Olin J, Schneider L | Galantamine for Alzheimer's disease | 2001, *Issue* 1 | Dementia and Cognitive Improvement |
| 40. Jepson RG, Kleijnen J, Leng GC | Garlic for peripheral arterial occlusive disease | 1997, *Issue* 3 | Peripheral Vascular Diseases |
| 41. Towheed TE, Anastassiades TP, Shea B, Houpt J, Welch V, Hochberg MC | Glucosamine therapy for osteoarthritis | 2001, *Issue* 1 | Musculoskeletal |
| 42. Evans JR | *Ginkgo biloba* extract for age-related macular degeneration | 1999, *Issue* 3 | Eyes and Vision |
| 43. Wilson ML, Murphy PA | Herbal and dietary therapies for primary and secondary dysmenorrhoea | 2001, *Issue* 3 | Menstrual Disorders and Subfertility |
| 44. Little CV, Parsons T | Herbal therapy for treating osteoarthritis | 2001, *Issue* 1 | Musculoskeletal |
| 45. Little C, Parsons T | Herbal therapy for treating rheumatoid arthritis | 2001, *Issue* 1 | Musculoskeletal |

| | Author | Title | Year | Group |
|---|---|---|---|---|
| 46. | Smith CA | Homeopathy for induction of labor | 2001, *Issue 4* | Pregnancy and Childbirth |
| 47. | Linde K, Jobst KA | Homeopathy for chronic asthma | 1998, *Issue 3* | Airways |
| 48. | Pittler MH, Ernst EE | Horse chestnut seed extract for chronic venous insufficiency | 2002, *Issue 1* | Peripheral Vascular Diseases |
| 49. | Vickers AJ, Smith C | Homoeopathic Oscillococcinum for preventing and treating influenza and influenza-like syndromes | 1999, *Issue 4* | Acute Respiratory Infections |
| 50. | Abbot NC, Stead LF, White AR, Barnes J, Ernst E | Hypnotherapy for smoking cessation | 1998, *Issue 2* | Tobacco and Addiction |
| 51. | Roberts L, Ahmed I, Hall S | Intercessory prayer for the alleviation of ill health | 1999, *Issue 1* | Schizophrenia |
| 52. | Jewell D, Young G | Interventions for nausea and vomiting in early pregnancy | 1996, *Issue 4* | Pregnancy and Childbirth |
| 53. | Campbell K, Waters E, O'Meara S, Summerbell C | Interventions for treating obesity in children | 2001, *Issue 1* | Heart Group |
| 54. | Bent S, Tsourinas C, Romoli M, Linde K | Kava for anxiety disorder | 2001, *Issue 4* | Depression, Anxiety, and Neurosis |
| 55. | Flemming K, Cullum N | Laser therapy for venous leg ulcers | 1998, *Issue 4* | Wounds |
| 56. | Higgins JPT, Flicker L | Lecithin for dementia and cognitive impairment | 2000, *Issue 2* | Dementia and Cognitive Improvement |
| 57. | Brosseau L, Welch V, Wells G, deBie R, Gam A, Harman K, Morin M, Shea B, Tugwell P | Low level laser therapy for OA [osteoarthritis] | 2000, *Issue 4* | Musculoskeletal |

Continued

## TABLE AI–1 Cochrane Reviews in Complementary Medicine—cont'd

| | AUTHORS | REVIEW TITLE | YEAR-ISSUE OR AMENDMENT | COCHRANE COLLABORATIVE REVIEW GROUP |
|---|---|---|---|---|
| 58. | Brosseau L, Welch V, Wells G, deBie R, Gam A, Harman K, Morin M, Shea B, Tugwell P | Low level laser therapy for RA [rheumatoid arthritis] | 2000, *Issue* 4 | Musculoskeletal |
| 59. | Rowe BH, Bretzlaff JA, Bourdon C, Bota GW, Camargo Jr CA | Magnesium sulfate for treating exacer-bations of acute asthma in the emer-gency department | 2000, *Issue* 4 | Airways |
| 60. | Hondras MA, Linde K, Jones AP | Manual therapy for asthma | 2000, *Issue* 3 | Airways |
| 61. | Furlan AD, Brosseau L, Welch V, Wong J | Massage for low back pain | 2000, *Issue* 4 | Back |
| 62. | Vickers A, Ohlsson A, Lacy JB, Horsley A | Massage to promote development in preterm and/or low birth weight infants | 1998, *Issue* 3 | Neonatal |
| 63. | Lui JP, Manheimer E, Tsutani K, Gluud C | Medicinal herbs for hepatitis C infection | 2001, *Issue* 4 | Hepato–Biliary |
| 64. | Herxheimer A, Petrie KJ | Melatonin for preventing and treating jet lag | 2001, *Issue* 1 | Depression, Anxiety, and Neurosis |
| 65. | Koger SM, Brotons M | Music therapy in dementia | 2001, *Issue* 1 | Dementia and Cognitive Improvement |
| 66. | Ferreira IM, Brooks D, Lacasse Y, Goldstein RS | Nutritional supplementation in stable chronic obstructive pulmonary disease | 2000, *Issue* 2 | Airways |
| 67. | Wilkinson EAJ, Hawke CI | Oral zinc for arterial and venous leg ulcers | 1998, *Issue* 3 | Wounds |
| 68. | Ram FSF, Robinson SM, Black PN | Physical training for asthma | 1999, *Issue* 1 | Airways |
| 69. | Wilt T, Ishani A, MacDonald R, Rutks I, Stark G | *Pygeum africanum* for benign prostatic hyperplasia | 2002, *Issue* 1 | Prostatic Diseases |

| | | | |
|---|---|---|---|
| 70. | Joy CB, Mumby-Croft R, Joy LA | Polyunsaturated fatty acid supplementation (fish or evening primrose oil) for schizophrenia | 2000, *Issue* 1 | Schizophrenia |
| 71. | Rambaldi A, Gluud C | S-adenosyl-L-methionine for alcoholic liver diseases | 2001, *Issue* 4 | Hepato-Biliary |
| 72. | Wilt T, Ishani A, Stark G, MacDonald R, Mulrow C, Lau J | *Serenoa repens* (saw palmetto) for benign prostatic hyperplasia | 1998, *Issue* 4 | Prostatic Diseases and Urological Disorders |
| 73. | Beamon S, Falkenbach A, Fainburg G, Linde K | Speleotherapy for the treatment of asthma | 2000, *Issue* 1 | Airways |
| 74. | Wilson ML, Murphy PA, Johnson TC, Farquhar CM | Spinal manipulation for primary and secondary dysmenorrhoea | 2001, *Issue* 4 | Menstrual Disorders and Subfertility |
| 75. | Linde K, Mulrow CD | St. John's wort for depression | 1998, *Issue* 2 | Depression, Anxiety, and Neurosis |
| 76. | Suresh GK, Davis JM, Soll RF | Superoxide dismutase for preventing chronic lung disease in mechanically ventilated preterm infants | 2001, *Issue* 1 | Neonatal |
| 77. | Carroll D, Moore RA, McQuay HJ, Fairman F, Tramer M, Leijon G | Transcutaneous nerve stimulation (TENS) for chronic pain | 2001 *Issue* 3 | Pain, Palliative Care, and Supportive Care |
| 78. | Proctor ML, Smith CA, Farquhar CM, Stones RW | Transcutaneous electrical nerve stimulation and acupuncture for primary dysmenorrhoea | 2001, *Issue* 1 | Pregnancy and Childbirth |
| 79. | Renfrew MJ, Lang S, Martin L, Woolridge MW | Treatments to relieve breast engorgement (previous review title: Cabbage leaves for breast engorgement) | 1999, *Issue* 4 | Pregnancy and Childbirth |
| 80. | Welch V, Brosseau L, Perterson J, Shea B, Tugwell P, Wells G | Therapeutic ultrasound for osteoarthritis of the knee | 2001, *Issue* 3 | Musculoskeletal |

*Continued*

**TABLE AI-1** Cochrane Reviews in Complementary Medicine—cont'd

| | AUTHORS | REVIEW TITLE | YEAR-ISSUE OR AMENDMENT | COCHRANE COLLABORATIVE REVIEW GROUP |
|---|---|---|---|---|
| 81. | Brosseau L, Casimiro L, Robinsinson V, Milne S, Shea B, Judd M, Wells G Tugwell, P | Therapeutic ultrasound for treating patellofemoral pain | 2001, *Issue* 4 | Musculoskeletal |
| 82. | Robinson V, Brosseau L, Casimiro L, Judd M, Shea B, Wells G, Tugwell P | Thermotherapy for treating rheumatoid arthritis | 2002, *Issue* 1 | Musculoskeletal |
| 83. | Shaw K, Turner J, Del Mar C | Trytophan and 5-hydroxytrytophan for depression | 2001, *Issue* 3 | Depression, Anxiety, and Neurosis |
| 84. | Van der Windt D, Van der Heijden GJMG, Van den Berg SGM | Ultrasound therapy for acute ankle sprains | 2001, *Issue* 4 | Musculoskeletal |
| 85. | Kaur B | Vitamin C supplementation for asthma | 2001, *Issue* 4 | Airways |
| 86. | Douglas RM, Chalker EB, Treacy B | Vitamin C for preventing and treating the common cold | 1998, *Issue* 1 | Acute Respiratory Infections |
| 87. | Kleijnen J, Mackerras D | Vitamin E for intermittent claudication | 1996, *Issue* 2 | Peripheral Vascular Diseases |
| 88. | Soares KVS, McGrath JJ | Vitamin E for neuroleptic-induced tardive dyskinesia | 2000, *Issue* 3 | Schizophrenia |
| 89. | Tabet N, Birks J, Grimley Evans J, Orrel M, Spector A | Vitamin E in Alzheimer's disease | 2000, *Issue* 4 | Dementia and Cognitive Improvement |
| 90. | Ramaratnam S, Sridharan K | Yoga in the treatment of epilepsy | 1999, *Issue* 3 | Epilepsy |
| 91. | Marshall I | Zinc in the treatment of the common cold | 1999, *Issue* 2 | Acute Respiratory Infections |
| 92. | Mahomed K | Zinc supplementation in pregnancy | 1997, *Issue* 3 | Pregnancy and Childbirth |

## TABLE AI-2 Cochrane Protocols In Complementary Medicine

| AUTHORS | PROTOCOL TITLE | YEAR–ISSUE OR AMENDMENT | COCHRANE COLLABORATIVE REVIEW GROUP |
|---|---|---|---|
| 1. Lee A, Done, ML | Acupoint P6 stimulation for preventing nausea and vomiting | 2001, *Issue 4* | Anesthesia |
| 2. Liu M, He L, Wu B, Zhang S, Asplund K | Acupuncture for acute stroke | 2001, *Issue 4* | Stroke Group |
| 3. He L, Zhou D, Wu B, Li N | Acupuncture for Bell's palsy | 2001, *Issue 1* | Neuromuscular Disease |
| 4. Richardson MA, Allen C, Ezzo J, Lao L, Ramirez G, Ramirez T, Zhang G | Acupuncture for chemotherapy-induced nausea or vomiting among cancer patients | 2000, *Issue 1* | Pain, Palliative Care, and Supportive Care |
| 5. Ezzo J, Hadhazy V, Berman B, Birch S, Kaplan G, Hochberg M | Acupuncture for osteoarthritis | 1998, *Issue 3* | Musculoskeletal |
| 6. Correia M, Veloso M, Correia C | Antioxidants for acute stroke | 1998, *Issue 3* | Stroke |
| 7. Correia M, Silva C, Veloso M | Antioxidants for secondary prevention after stroke/transient ischaemic attack | 1999, *Issue 3* | Stroke |
| 8. Orrell RW, Lane RJM, Ross M | Antioxidant treatment for amyotrophic lateral sclerosis/motor neuron disease | 2001, *Issue 1* | Neuromuscular Disease |
| 9. Hooper L, Capps N, Clements G, Davey Smith G, Ebrahim S, Higgins J, Ness A, Riemersma RA, Summerbell CD | Antioxidant foods or supplements for preventing cardiovascular disease | 1999, *Issue 2* | Heart Group |
| 10. Thorgrimsen L, Spector A, Orrell M, Wiles A | Aroma therapy for dementia | 2001, *Issue 3* | Dementia and Cognitive Improvement |
| 11. Ruddy R, Milnes D | Art therapy for schizophrenia/ schizophrenia-like illnesses | 2002, *Issue 3* | Schizophrenia |
| 12. Wilson ML, Murphy PA, Pattison HM, Farquhar CM | Behavioural interventions for primary and secondary dysmenorrhoea | 2000, *Issue 3* | Menstrual Disorders and Infertility |

Continued

# TABLE AI-2 Cochrane Protocols In Complementary Medicine—cont'd

| AUTHORS | PROTOCOL TITLE | YEAR-ISSUE OR AMENDMENT | COCHRANE COLLABORATIVE REVIEW GROUP |
|---|---|---|---|
| 13. Hoare C, Leonard T, Williams HC | Chinese herbal medicine for atopic eczema | 2000, *Issue* 2 | Skin |
| 14. Hoare C, Leonard T, Williams HC | Chinese medicinal herbs for asymptomatic carriers of hepatitis B | 2000, *Issue* 3 | Hepato-Biliary |
| 15. Charlesworth G, Riordan J, Shepstone L | Cognitive behavior therapy for depressed caregivers of people with Alzheimer's disease and related disorders | 1999, *Issue* 4 | Dementia and Cognitive Improvement |
| 16. Coates P, Eady AE, Cove JH | Complementary therapies for acne | 1999, *Issue* 2 | Skin |
| 17. Caraballoso M, Bonfill X, Serra C | Drugs for preventing lung cancer | 2000, *Issue* 1 | Lung Cancer |
| 18. Ruether A, Bueschel G, Leipner J, Linde K, Rostock M, Horneber M | Enzyme therapy in oncology | 2000, *Issue* 4 | Gynaecological Cancer Group |
| 19. Makrides M, Duley L, Olsen SF | Fish oil and other prostaglandin precursor supplementation during pregnancy for reducing preterm birth, pre-eclampsia, low birth weight, and in-trauterine growth restriction | 2001, *Issue* 4 | Pregnancy and Childbirth |
| 20. Strid J, Jepson R, Moore V, Kleijnen J, Iasco SM | Evening primrose oil or other essential fatty acids for premenstrual syndrome | 1998, *Issue* 2 | Menstrual Disorders and Subfertility |
| 21. Taylor M, Carney S, Geddes J, Goodwin G | Folate for depressive disorders | 2001, *Issue* 4 | Depression, Anxiety, and Neurosis |
| 22. Ness A, Hooper L, Egger M, Powles JW, Davey Smith G | Fruits and vegetables for cardiovascular disease | 2001, *Issue* 4 | Heart Group |
| 23. Zeng X, Lui M, Asplund K, Yang Y, Zhang S, Wu B | *Ginkgo biloba* for acute ischaemic stroke | 2003, *Issue* 3 | Stroke |
| 24. Kleijnen J | *Ginkgo biloba* for intermittent claudication | 1996, *Issue* 2 | Peripheral Vascular Diseases |

| 25. | Novak F, Avenell A, Heyland DK, Croal BL, Drover JW, Jain M, Noble D, Su X | Glutamine supplementation for critically ill adults | 2000, *Issue* 3 | Anesthesia |
| 26. | Liu JP, Yang M, Du XM | Herbal medicines for viral myocarditis | 2003, *Issue* 3 | Infectious Disease |
| 27. | Bent S, Tsourinas C, Romoli M, Linde K | Kava for anxiety disorder | 1999, *Issue* 3 | Depression, Anxiety, and Neurosis |
| 28. | Beamon S, Falkenbach A, Jobst K | Hydrotherapy for asthma | 1999, *Issue* 4 | Airways |
| 29. | Gross AR, Hondras MA, Aker PD, Peloso P, Goldsmith CH | Manual therapy for mechanical neck disorders | 1997, *Issue* 3 | Back |
| 30. | Lockhart-Wood K, Gambles M, Wilkinson S | Massage and aromatherapy for symptom relief in patients with cancer | 2000, *Issue* 3 | Pain, Palliative Care, and Supportive Care |
| 31. | Liu JP, Manheimer E, Tsutani K, Gluud C | Medicinal herbs for hepatitis C virus infection | 2001, *Issue* 4 | Hepato-Biliary |
| 32. | Liu JP, Gluud C | Medicinal herbs vs medicinal herbs for chronic hepatitis B virus infection | 2001, *Issue* 3 | Hepato-Biliary |
| 33. | Hadhazy V, Ezzo JM, Berman BM, Creamer P, Bausell B | Mind/body therapy for fibromyalgia | 2000, *Issue* 3 | Musculoskeletal |
| 34. | Horneber MA, Bueschel G, Huber R, Linde K, Richardson MA, Rostock M, Kaiser G | Mistletoe therapy in oncology | 2001, *Issue* 4 | Gynaecological Cancer |
| 35. | Bronfort G, Nilsson N, Assendelft WJJ, Bouter LM, Goldsmith C, Evans R, Haas M | Noninvasive physical treatments for chronic headache | 1999, *Issue* 3 | Pain, Palliative Care, and Supportive Care |
| 36. | Langer G, Scholoemer G, Lautenschlaeger C | Nutrition for preventing and treating pressure ulcers | 2001, *Issue* 3 | Wounds |
| 37. | Hooper L, Thompson R, Harrison R, Summerbell C, Higgins J | Omega-3 fatty acids for prevention of cardiovascular disease | 2001, *Issue* 3 | Heart Group |
| 38. | Beckles Willson N, Elliott TM, Everard ML | Omega-3 fatty acids for cystic fibrosis | 2000, *Issue* 3 | Cystic Fibrosis and Genetic Disorders |
| 39. | Juni P, Fux C, Hertog MGL, Egger M, Ernst E | Padma 28 (a Tibetan herbal preparation) for intermittent claudication | 1997, *Issue* 4 | Peripheral Vascular Diseases |

*Continued*

## TABLE AI-2 Cochrane Protocols In Complementary Medicine—cont'd

| AUTHORS | PROTOCOL TITLE | YEAR-ISSUE OR AMENDMENT | COCHRANE COLLABORATIVE REVIEW GROUP |
|---|---|---|---|
| 40. Greener J, Enderby P, Whurr R | Pharmacological treatment for aphasia following stroke | 1998, *Issue 2* | Stroke |
| 41. Lethaby AE, Kronenberg F, Roberts H, Eden J | Phytoestrogens for menopausal symptoms | 1998, *Issue 4* | Menstrual Disorders and Subfertility |
| 42. Ardila E, Echevery J | Phytoestrogens in the treatment of postmenopausal osteoporosis | 2001, *Issue 3* | Musculoskeletal |
| 43. Gambles MA, Lockhart-Wood K, Wilkinson SM | Reflexology for symptom relief in patients with cancer | 2001, *Issue 1* | Prostatic Diseases |
| 44. Darlow BA, Austin NC | Selenium supplementation to prevent short-term morbidity in preterm neonates | 2001, *Issue 4* | Neonatal |
| 45. Assendeift WJJ, Shekelle PG | Spinal manipulation for low back pain | 1996, *Issue 1* | Back |
| 46. Rees K, Bennett P, Vedhara K, West R, Davey Smith G, Ebrahim S | Stress management for coronary heart disease | 2001, *Issue 1* | Heart Group |
| 47. Martin JLR, Barbanoj MJ, Clos S | Transcranial magnetic stimulation for the treatment of depression | 2001, *Issue 4* | Depression, Anxiety, and Neurosis |
| 48. Martin JLR, Barbanoj MJ, Clos S | Transcranial magnetic stimulation for the treatment of obsessive compulsive disorder | 2001, *Issue 4* | Depression, Anxiety, and Neurosis |
| 49. O'Mathuna D | Therapeutic Touch in wound healing | 1998, *Issue 3* | Wounds |
| 50. Iasco SM, Castro AA, Atallah AN | Vitamin B$_6$ and placebo in premenstrual syndrome | 1998, *Issue 4* | Menstrual Disorders and Subfertility |

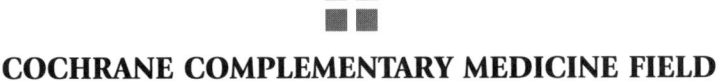

# COCHRANE COMPLEMENTARY MEDICINE FIELD

In 1996, to meet the tremendous need for high-quality information in complementary medicine, the Complementary Medicine Field was established to help promote and facilitate the production of systematic reviews on topics such as acupuncture, massage, chiropractic, herbal medicine, homeopathy, and mind-body therapy. The activities of the field include maintaining and updating the CM registry of trials (randomized controlled and clinical controlled trials), assisting reviewers doing CM reviews, providing references for all Cochrane Collaboration CM reviews, maintaining a registry of reviews, and refining literature search strategies for identifying CM literature.

The field works with the appropriate CRG to write systematic reviews. The research question determines which of the CRGs works with the field for a specific review. For example, whether massage is effective for increasing the weight of low birth weight infants was done in collaboration with the neonatal CRG. The effectiveness of mind-body therapy for fibromyalgia was done with the musculoskeletal CRG. This collaborative effort ensures that every systematic review receives input from practitioners who perform that treatment, scientists who are experts in research methodology, specialists who are experts in the disease under study, and consumers who represent the viewpoint of the patient and lay public.

The central coordinating body of the Complementary Medicine Field is currently a 15-member advisory board consisting of methodologists and clinicians from a variety of CM backgrounds in eight countries. Individual positions such as field coordinator, field administrator, and registry coordinator also provide for the performance of specific field functions. The field coordinator for CM currently is Brian Berman, M.D., of the University of Maryland in Baltimore, Maryland. Dr. Berman chairs the advisory board, and his role is to promote the perspectives and priorities of the field within and outside the Cochrane Collaboration. He regularly informs the Cochrane Centers and Steering Committee of the present endeavors and future plans of the field.

The current registry coordinator, Mac Beckner of the Complementary Medicine Program at the University of Maryland at Baltimore, fulfills the function of identifying reports of clinical trials and making them accessible. To this end he maintains the specialized CM database. CISCOM (the database of the Research Council of Complementary Medicine in London) provided much of the original data for the CM registry. Other sources of information include databases such as MEDLINE and EMBASE and hand-searched sources such as complementary medicine journals, conference proceedings, and dissertations as well as contact with researchers in the field. Because some of these studies are unpublished, a paper copy archive presently is being developed. Finally, to reduce publication bias, the registry coordinator establishes a trials registry of ongoing and planned CM trials.

The principal external institution with which the field has established affiliation is the NIH National Center for Complementary and Alternative Medicine. NCCAM supports the efforts of the CM Field by providing funding and creating scientific forums by which research issues in complementary medicine can be discussed. Other external links internationally include persons and organizations that offer their skills and time to assist with systematic reviews in their areas of competence, hand search journals from their respective countries, or retrieve studies for the complementary medicine database.

## REGISTRY OF TRIALS

The CM Field has put a great deal of effort into laying the groundwork for conducting reviews by constructing a database of randomized controlled trials (RCTs) and clinical controlled trials (CCTs) on complementary and alternative medicine topics. To date, more than 5800 trials have been identified through regular high-yield search strategies (Fig. AI-1). Aside from electronic searches, members of the CM Field regularly hand search more than 40 high-priority journals. On a quarterly basis, the CM registry uploads its trials to the Cochrane Controlled Trials Registry, making these trials available to individuals with access to the Cochrane Library. The registry is also available on the Complementary Medicine Field Web site.

## REGISTRY OF REVIEWS

In addition to the registry of trials, the CM Field maintains a database of Cochrane reviews and a database of non-Cochrane reviews. Through the combination of these efforts more than 230 reviews have been identified in CM, including 80 Cochrane reviews. Conducting systematic reviews in complementary medicine is a unique and often time-consuming process primarily because much of the research literature is scattered among many online and print sources. The CM registry brings this literature together in one easily accessible place for researchers, consumers, and practitioners.

## MEDICAL SUBJECT HEADINGS

Additional challenges to conducting reviews include inconsistencies in how complementary medicine is defined and indexed by leading biomedical databases. For example, Chinese movement therapies such as *qi gong* and *tai chi* are considered complementary therapies by the standards of the field but are not accessed by a

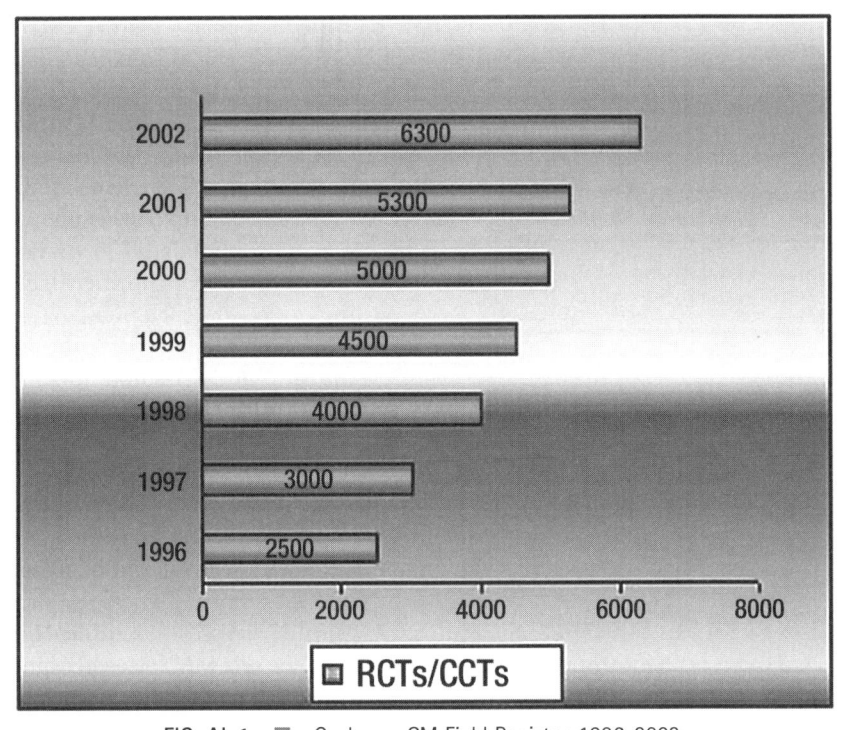

FIG. AI-1   ■   Cochrane CM Field Registry, 1996-2002.

hierarchical MEDLINE search of the MeSH term *"alternative medicine."* Herbal remedies may be described by MEDLINE as plant extracts rather than by any alternative
medicine term. To aid MEDLINE searching, the field has assisted in creating a comprehensive MEDLINE search strategy that is now available for public use.

## COMPLETED REVIEWS

To date, over 90 CM-related systematic reviews are published in the Cochrane Library
and approximately 46 more are under way (Fig. AI-2). In addition to gathering randomized controlled trials of complementary medicine, CM Field members are also
tracking down and assessing systematic reviews. In 1998 field members began a project to review the quality of CM reviews. This project has resulted in the publication
of three landmark systematic reviews on BioMed Central covering acupuncture,
homeopathy, and herbal medicine. In the course of these reviews, nearly 150 systematic reviews were evaluated and 115 met inclusion criteria. Reviews such as these are
invaluable for identifying and addressing not only the efficacy of CM therapies but
also the methodological and research design issues.

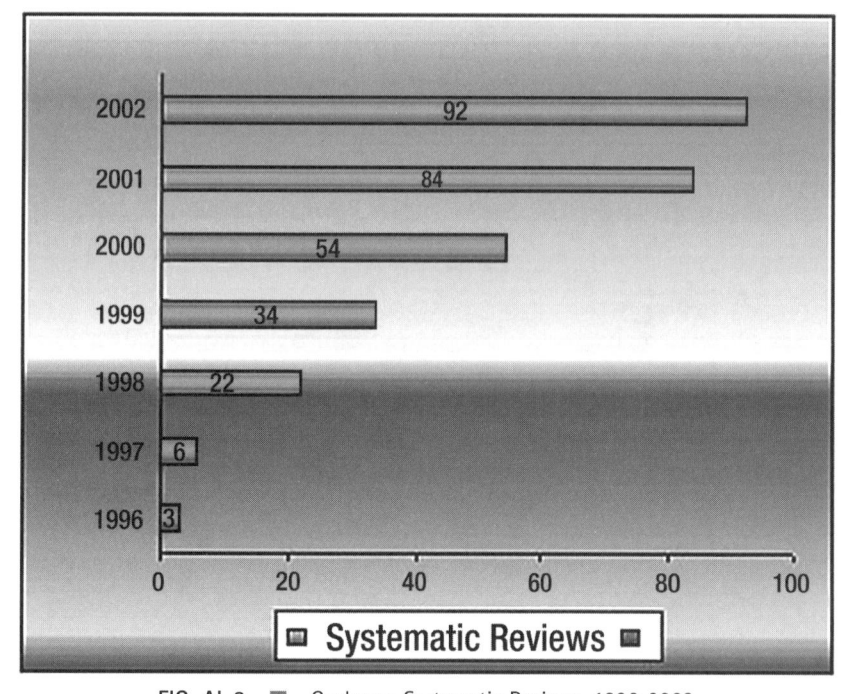

FIG. AI-2  ■  Cochrane Systematic Reviews, 1996-2002.

Recently, Cochrane CM reviews have provided a reliable basis for making health care decisions. For example, the Cochrane systematic review of St. John's wort (*Hypericum perforatum*) for mild to moderate depression included 27 trials with a total of more than 2000 participants. The review found that St. John's wort was superior to placebo and equivalent to tricyclic antidepressants but had fewer adverse effects. Although not all questions have been answered, particularly those of safety, the review does provide a basis for making treatment decisions. Additionally, a recent CM review examined the effects of saw palmetto (*Serenoa repens*) on benign prostatic hyperplasia. Eighteen studies with a total sample size of nearly 3000 patients were included. Clear benefits were shown for urinary symptoms and peak urine flow. Other recent, high-quality systematic reviews (not all Cochrane reviews) have found acupuncture to be effective for pain and nausea but not for helping smokers to quit. To a greater extent these reviews are a reflection of the rapid growth in applied research in CM. A key element in this growth has been the dramatic increase in research funding combined with the application of evidence-based methodologies in the evaluation and dissemination of high-quality systematic reviews in CM.

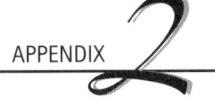

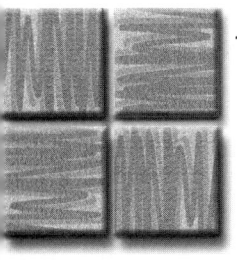

APPENDIX 2

# Continuing Medical Education in Complementary and Alternative Medicine

## CONTINUING MEDICAL EDUCATION COURSES

A number of organizations, primarily academic medical schools, offer continuing medical education (CME) courses in complementary medicine:

**Columbia University College of Physicians & Surgeons**
CME: Botanical Medicine in Modern Clinical Practice
Fredi Kronenberg
Center for Continuing Education
630 West 168th Street, Unit 39
New York, NY 10032
(212) 781-5990
cme@columbia.edu
http://cpmcnet.columbia.edu/dept/cme

**Columbia University College of Physicians & Surgeons**
CME: Integrative Pain Medicine
James N. Dillard, M.D., and Fredi Kronenberg, Ph.D.
Department of Rehabilitation Medicine
The Richard and Hilda Rosenthal Center for Complementary & Alternative Medicine
http://www.rosenthal.hs.columbia.edu/integ_pain.html

**George Washington University**
CME: Primary Care for the 21st Century: Holistic Medicine
American Holistic Medical Association
6728 Old McLean Village Drive
McLean, VA 22101
(703) 556-9245

**Harvard Medical School**
CME: Alternative Medicine: Implications for Clinical Practice
Norman Shostak
Harvard Medical School, CME
641 Huntington Avenue
Boston, MA 02215
(617) 432-0196, (617) 432-1562 (fax)
nshostak@warren.med.harvard.edu

**Harvard Medical School**
CME: Clinical Training in Mind/Body Medicine
Herbert Benson, M.D.
Harvard Medical School, CME
641 Huntington Avenue
Boston, MA 02215
(617) 432-1525
hms-cme@warren.med.harvard.edu

**Rush Medical College**
CME: Annual Mind-Body Medicine Conference
William Schwer, M.D.
Department of Family Medicine
Rush-Presbyterian–St. Luke's Medical Center
600 South Paulina, Suite 749
Chicago, IL 60612
(312) 942-7083

**University of Arizona School of Medicine**
Program in Integrative Medicine
Andrew Weil, M.D.
Department of Medicine, Box 245153
Tucson, AZ 85724-5153
(520) 626-5077, (520) 626-2757 (fax)

**University of California, Los Angeles, School of Medicine**
CME: Medical Acupuncture for Physicians
Joseph M. Helms, M.D.
2520 Milvia Street
Berkeley, CA 94704
(510) 649-8488, (510) 649-8692 (fax)

**University of California, Los Angeles, School of Medicine**
CME: Integrative East-West Medicine
Ka Kit Hui, M.D., FACP
200 UCLA Medical Plaza
Suite 420
Los Angeles, CA 90095
(310) 206-1895, (310) 794-1896 (fax)

**University of Colorado Health Sciences Center**
CME: The Scientific Basis for Using Holistic Medicine to Treat Chronic Disease
Robert S. Ivker, D.O., and Louise Kosenski
A.F. Williams Family Medicine Center
5250 Leetsdale Drive, Suite 304
Denver, CO 80222
(303) 388-0965, ext. 108

**University of Massachusetts Medical School**
  CME: Evidence-Based Botanical Medicine
  Cambridge Health Resources
  1037 Chestnut Street
  Newton, MA 02464
  (617) 630-1330, (617) 630-1325 (fax)
**University of Minnesota—Minneapolis**
  CMEs: Complementary Care: From Principles to Practice and The Scientific Basis
    for the Holistic Treatment of Chronic Disease
  William Manahan, M.D.
  University of Minnesota CME
  308 Harvard Street SE, Suite 6-101
  Minneapolis, MN 55455
  (800) 776-8636, (612) 626-4772
  (612) 626-7766 (fax)
**University of New Mexico School of Medicine**
  CME: Alternative Medicine
  Martin Kantrowitz, M.D., and Lee Stephenson
  Office of CME, Box 517
  Albuquerque, NM 87131
  (505) 277-6611, (505) 277-7087 (fax)
  lstephen@medusa.unm.edu
**University of Vermont College of Medicine**
  CME: The Scientific Basis for Using Holistic Medicine to Treat Chronic Disease
  Richard B. White, M.D.
  Family Practice Health Care Service
  Office of Continuing Medical Education
  One South Prospect Street
  Burlington, VT 05401-3444
  (802) 656-2292
**Wayne State University School of Medicine**
  CME: A Course in Clinical Hypnosis: Basic Level
  Marilyn P. Laken, Ph.D., R.N.
  Department of OB/GYN, Hutzel Hospital
  4707 St. Antoine
  Detroit, MI 48201
  (313) 577-1147, (313) 577-2045 (fax)
  mlaken@med.wayne.edu

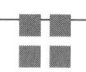

# FELLOWSHIPS AND RESIDENCY TRAINING

The number of fellowships available has been expanded to stimulate the development of CAM research, not simply by funding clinical studies but also by supporting the professional development of researchers. Several major medical schools are now providing postdoctoral fellowships relevant to research in complementary medicine.

**Emory University School of Medicine**
> Post-Doctoral Fellowship in Complementary and Alternative Medicine (CAM) in Movement Disorders, Department of Neurology, Georgia Institute of Technology Center for Human Movement Studies
> Charles M. Epstein, M.D.
> Associate Professor of Neurology
> Department of Neurology
> 1365 Clifton Road, NE
> Atlanta, GA 30322
> (404) 778-3633, (404) 778-3767 (fax)
> http://www.emory.edu/WHSC/MED/NEUROLOGY/CAM/POSTDOCFELLOLINK.htm

**Harvard Medical School**
> Center for Alternative Medicine Research and Education
> Faculty Development and Fellowship Program in CAM
> Division of General Medicine
> Beth Israel Deaconess Medical Center
> 330 Brookline Avenue, Libby-330
> Boston, MA 02215
> http://www.bidmc.harvard.edu/medicine/camr/Whatsnew.html

**Montefiore Medical Center**
> Residency Program in Social Medicine
> Ellen Tattleman, M.D.
> Valentine Lane Family Practice
> 503 South Broadway
> Bronx, NY 10705
> (914) 965-9771

**Oregon Health and Science University**
> The Oregon Center for Complementary and Alternative Medicine (OCCAM)
> OCCAM Post-Doctoral Research Fellowship
> A cooperative 2-year fellowship among six health care institutions in Portland
> Katherine J. Riley, Ed.D.
> Public Health and Preventive Medicine
> OHSU
> 3181 S.W. Sam Jackson Park Road, CB 669
> Portland, OR 97201-309
> http://www.ohsu.edu/som-PubHealth/postdoc.html

**University of Arizona School of Medicine**
Fellowship, Program in Integrative Medicine
Andrew Weil, M.D., and Victoria Maizes, M.D.
Department of Medicine
PO Box 245-153
Tucson, AZ 85724-5153
(520) 626-5077
http://integrativemedicine.arizona.edu/fellowship.html

**University of Maryland School of Medicine**
Fellowship in Pain/Complementary Medicine
Brian Berman, M.D.
Complementary Medicine Program
Kernan Hospital Mansion
2200 Kernan Drive
Baltimore, MD 21207-6697
(410) 448-6872
http://www.compmed.umm.edu/

---

# PROFESSIONAL TRAINING

**Botanicals for Women's Health**
*UIC/NIH Center for Botanical Dietary Supplement Research in Women's Health*
This online program provides pharmacists and other allied health professionals with an understanding of the therapeutic uses, mechanism(s) of action, contraindications, adverse or potentially adverse reactions, drug interactions, dose and dosage forms for some of the most popular botanical dietary supplements associated with women's health. The program is accredited by the American Council on Pharmaceutical Education
http://www.uic.edu/pharmacy/conted/botanicals/

**Current Issues in Dietary Supplements**
*University of Florida, College of Agricultural and Life Sciences, Institute of Food and Agricultural Life Sciences, Department of Food Science and Human Nutrition*
This course introduces federal laws and regulations covering the definitions, marketing, and labeling of dietary supplements. Discussion focuses on specific vitamins, minerals, herbs, and ergogenic aids. Review of scientific literature and public information is provided.
Academic credits: 2 graduate credits
http://grove.ufl.edu/%7Ehun5246

### Herbal Medicine
*American Botanical Council*

A course approved by the American Dietetic Association (ADA) is offered through the American Botanical Council and University of Texas School of Pharmacy and contains comprehensive monographs for 29 herbs, a clinical overview with clinical studies table, and patient information sheets for copying and distribution. Course is available after June 2002. For more information about 2003 course offerings, contact *continuinged@herbalgram.org.*

### Hypnosis
Course in Clinical Hypnosis: Basic Level
Marilyn Laken, Ph.D., R.N.
Department of OB/GYN, Hutzel Hospital
4707 St. Antoine
Detroit, MI 48201
(313) 577-2045

### Mind-Body Medicine
Clinical Training in Mind-Body Medicine
Herbert Benson, M.D.
Harvard Medical School
641 Huntington Avenue
Boston, MA 02215
(617) 432-1525
http://www.mbmi.org/pages/tfhp_ut2.asp

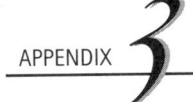

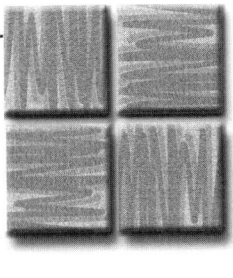

# Glossary of Complementary and Alternative Medicine Terms

**Acupressure:** Based on the principles of acupuncture, this ancient Chinese technique involves using finger pressure on specific points along the body to treat ailments.

**Acupuncture:** This therapy is used to relieve pain, improve well-being, and treat acute, chronic, and degenerative conditions in children and adults. In Asian medicine, acupuncture needles are inserted at specific points to stimulate, disperse, and regulate the flow of *chi*, or vital energy, and restore a healthy energy balance.

**Alexander technique:** This therapeutic technique aims to use efficiently movement and posture to improve health and reduce pain.

**Anthroposophic medicine:** Developed by philosopher and mystic Rudolf Steiner (1861-1925), this medical system takes into account the spiritual and physical components of illness. A treatment regimen may include herbal and homeopathic medicines and dietary recommendations, art therapy, movement therapy, massage, and specially prepared baths.

**Aromatherapy:** This therapy uses essential oils (the volatile oils distilled from plants) to treat emotional disorders such as stress and anxiety and a wide range of other ailments. Oils are massaged into the skin, inhaled, or placed in baths. Aromatherapy often is used with massage therapy, acupuncture, reflexology, herbology, chiropractic, and other holistic treatments.

**Ayurvedic medicine:** Practiced in India for more than 5000 years, Ayurvedic tradition holds that illness is a state of imbalance among body systems that can be detected through diagnostic procedures such as reading the pulse and observing the tongue. Nutrition counseling, massage, natural medications, meditation, and other modalities are used to address a broad spectrum of diseases.

**Bioenergetics:** This philosophy holds that repressed emotions and desires affect the body and psyche by creating chronic muscular tension and diminished vitality and energy. Through physical exercises, breathing techniques, verbal psychotherapy, or other forms of emotional-release work, the therapist attempts to loosen the "character armor" and restore natural well-being.

**Biofeedback:** A technique used especially for stress-related conditions, such as asthma, migraines, insomnia, and high blood pressure, biofeedback is a way of monitoring minute metabolic changes in one's own body (for example, temperature changes, heart rate, and muscle tension) with the aid of sensitive machines. By consciously visualizing, relaxing, or imagining while observing light, sound, or metered feedback, the client learns to make subtle adjustments to move toward a more balanced internal state.

**Breathwork:** This general term describes a variety of techniques that use patterned breathing to promote physical, mental, and spiritual well-being. Some techniques use the breath in a calm, peaceful way to induce relaxation or manage pain, whereas others use stronger breathing to stimulate emotions and emotional release.

**Chelation therapy:** Typically administered in an osteopathic or medical doctor's office, chelation therapy is a series of intravenous injections of the synthetic amino acid ethylenediaminetetraacetic acid, designed to detoxify the body. The treatment often is used to treat arteriosclerosis, or hardening of the arteries.

**Chinese (Asian) medicine:** Asian medical practitioners are trained to use a variety of ancient and modern therapeutic methods—including acupuncture, herbal medicine, massage, moxibustion (heat therapy), and nutritional and lifestyle counseling—to treat a broad range of chronic and acute illnesses.

**Chiropractic:** The chiropractic system is based on the premise that the spine is literally the backbone of human health: misalignments of the vertebrae caused by poor posture or trauma result in pressure on the spinal cord, which may lead to diminished function and illness. The chiropractor seeks to analyze and correct these misalignments through spinal manipulation or adjustment.

**Craniosacral therapy:** A manual therapeutic procedure used to remedy distortions in the structure and function of the craniosacral mechanism: the brain and spinal cord, the bones of the skull, the sacrum, and interconnected membranes. The procedure is used to treat chronic pain, migraine headaches, temporomandibular joint disease, and a range of other conditions and is performed by a range of licensed health practitioners.

**Dance/movement therapies:** This therapy uses expressive movement as a therapeutic tool for personal expression and psychological or emotional healing. Practitioners work with individuals with physical disabilities, addictions, histories of sexual abuse, eating disorders, and other concerns.

**Deep tissue bodywork:** This general term describes a range of therapies for unsticking the connective tissues and muscles to encourage them to function properly again. Among the conditions deep tissue bodywork treats are whiplash, low back and neck pain, and degenerative diseases such as multiple sclerosis.

**Dentistry, holistic:** Holistic dentists are licensed dentists who bring an interdisciplinary approach to their practices, often incorporating methods such as homeopathy, nutrition, and acupuncture into their treatment plans. Most holistic dentists emphasize wellness and preventive care and avoid (and often recommend the removal of) silver-mercury fillings.

**Energy field work:** Practitioners of this range of therapies look for weaknesses in the person's energy field in and around the body and seek to restore its proper circulation and balance. Energy channeled through the practitioner is directed to strengthen the natural defenses of the body and help the person's physical, mental, emotional, and spiritual state. Sessions may or may not involve the physical laying-on of hands.

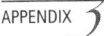 

**Feldenkrais:** This therapy combines movement training, gentle touch, and verbal dialogue to help create more efficient movement. In individual hands-on sessions, the practitioner's touch is used to address the student's breathing and body alignment along with a series of slow, nonaerobic motions.

**Feng shui:** Pronounced "fung shway," this is the ancient Chinese practice of configuring home or work environments to promote health, happiness, and prosperity. *Feng shui* consultants may advise clients to make adjustments in their surroundings—from color selection to furniture placement—to promote a healthy flow of *chi,* or vital energy.

**Flower essences:** Popularized by Edward Bach, M.D., flower essences are intended to alleviate negative emotional states that may contribute to illness or hinder personal growth. Drops of a solution infused with the captured essence of a flower are placed under the tongue or in a beverage. The practitioner helps the client choose appropriate essences, focusing on the client's emotional state rather than on a particular physical condition.

**Gestalt therapy:** This psychotherapy aims to help the client achieve wholeness (*gestalt* is the German word for whole) by becoming fully aware of his or her feelings, perceptions, and behavior. The emphasis is on immediate experience rather than on the past. Gestalt therapy often is conducted in group settings such as weekend workshops.

**Guided imagery:** This therapy involves using mental images to promote physical healing or changes in attitudes or behavior. Practitioners may lead clients through specific visualization exercises or offer instruction in using imagery as a self-help tool. Guided imagery often is used to alleviate stress and to treat stress-related conditions such as insomnia and high blood pressure. The therapy also is used by persons with cancer, AIDS, chronic fatigue syndrome, and other disorders with the aim of boosting the immune system.

**Healing touch:** Registered nurses and others practice this therapy to accelerate wound healing, relieve pain, promote relaxation, prevent illness, and ease the dying process. The practitioner uses light touch or works with his or her hands near the client's body in an effort to restore balance to the client's energy system.

**Herbalism:** An ancient form of healing still widely used in much of the world, herbalism uses natural plants or plant-based substances to treat a range of illnesses and to enhance the functioning of body systems. Though herbalism is not a licensed professional modality in the United States, herbs are "prescribed" by a range of practitioners, from holistic medical doctors to acupuncturists and naturopaths.

**Holistic medicine:** This broadly descriptive term describes a healing philosophy that views a patient as a whole person, not as just a disease or a collection of symptoms. In the course of treatment, holistic medical practitioners may address a client's emotional and spiritual dimensions and the nutritional, environmental, and lifestyle factors that may contribute to an illness.

**Homeopathy:** This medical system uses minute doses of natural substances—called *remedies*—to stimulate a person's immune and defense system. A remedy is chosen individually for a sick person based on its capacity to cause, if given in overdose, physical and psychological symptoms similar to those a patient is experiencing.

**Hypnotherapy:** The term describes a range of techniques that allow practitioners to bypass the conscious mind and access the subconscious, where suppressed memories, repressed emotions, and forgotten events may remain recorded. Hypnosis may facilitate behavioral, emotional, or attitudinal change.

**Iridology:** This diagnostic system is based on the premise that every organ has a corresponding location within the iris of the eye, which can serve as an indicator of the individual health or disease of an organ. Iridology is used by naturopaths and other practitioners, particularly when diagnosis achieved through standard methods is unclear.

**Kinesiology/applied kinesiology:** Kinesiology is the study of muscles and their movements. Applied kinesiology is a system that uses muscle testing procedures, with standard methods of diagnosis, to gain information about a patient's overall state of health. Practitioners analyze muscle function, posture, gait, and other structural factors in addition to inquiring about lifestyle factors that may be contributing to a health-related problem.

**Macrobiotic diet:** This diet consists of whole grains, vegetables, sea vegetables, and seeds. These natural foods, cooked in accordance with macrobiotic principles designed to synchronize eating habits with the cycles of nature, are used to promote health and minimize disease.

**Magnets:** Magnetic therapy (also known as *magnetic field therapy* or *biomagnetic therapy*) involves using magnets, magnetic devices, or magnetic fields to treat a variety of physical and emotional conditions, including circulatory problems, certain forms of arthritis, chronic pain, sleep disorders, and stress. Treatments may be applied by a practitioner or as part of a self-care program.

**Massage therapy:** This general term describes a range of therapeutic approaches with roots in Eastern and Western cultures. Massage therapy involves the practice of kneading or otherwise manipulating a person's muscles and other soft tissue with the intent of improving a person's well-being or health.

**Meditation:** This general term describes a wide range of practices that involve training one's attention or awareness so that body and mind can be brought into greater harmony. Although some meditators may seek a mystical sense of oneness with a higher power or with the universe, others may seek to reduce stress or alleviate stress-related ailments such as anxiety and high blood pressure.

**Myofascial release:** This hands-on technique seeks to free the body from the grip of tight fascia, or connective tissue, thus restoring normal alignment and function and reducing pain. Using their hands, therapists gently apply mild, sustained pressure to stretch and soften the fascia. Myofascial release is used to treat conditions such as neck and back pain, headaches, recurring sports injuries, and scoliosis.

**Naturopathic medicine:** This primary health care system emphasizes the curative power of nature and treats acute and chronic illnesses in all age groups. Naturopathic physicians work to restore and support the body's own healing ability using a variety of modalities including nutrition, herbal medicine, homeopathic medicine, and Asian medicine.

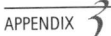

**Neuromuscular therapy:** This therapy emphasizes the role of the brain, spine, and nerves in muscular pain. One goal of the therapy is to relieve tender, congested spots in muscle tissue and compressed nerves that may radiate pain to other areas of the body.

**Nursing, holistic:** More a philosophy than a series of practices, holistic nursing is embraced by registered or licensed nurses who seek to care for the body, mind, and spirit of the patient. Some holistic nurses work in independent practices, offering primary and chronic care that incorporates a variety of alternative methods, from homeopathy to Therapeutic Touch.

**Osteopathic medicine:** Like medical doctors, osteopathic physicians provide comprehensive medical care, including preventive medicine, diagnosis, surgery, prescription medications, and hospital referrals. In diagnosis and treatment, they pay particular attention to the joints, bones, muscles, and nerves and are trained specially in osteopathic manipulative treatment—using their hands to diagnose, treat, and prevent illness.

**Qi gong (chi–kung):** This ancient Chinese exercise system aims to stimulate and balance the flow of *qi* (*chi*), or vital energy, along the acupuncture meridians, or energy pathways. *Qi gong* is used to reduce stress, improve blood circulation, enhance immune function, and treat a variety of health conditions.

**Reflexology:** This philosophy is based on the idea that specific points on the feet and hands correspond with organs and tissues throughout the body. With fingers and thumbs, the practitioner applies pressure to these points to treat a wide range of stress-related illnesses and ailments.

**Reiki:** Practitioners of this ancient Tibetan healing system use light hand placements to channel healing energies to the recipient. Although practitioners may vary widely in technique and philosophy, *reiki* commonly is used to treat emotional and mental distress and chronic and acute physical problems and to assist the recipient in achieving spiritual focus and clarity.

**Shiatsu:** The most widely known form of acupressure, *shiatsu* has been used in Japan for more than 1000 years to treat pain and illness and for general health maintenance. Using a series of techniques, practitioners apply rhythmic finger pressure at specific points on the body to stimulate *chi,* or vital energy.

**Spiritual/shamanic healing:** Practitioners of spiritual healing and shamanic healing often regard themselves as conductors of healing energy or sources from the spiritual realm. Both may call on spiritual helpers such as power animals (characteristic of the shaman), angels, inner teachers, the client's higher self, or other spiritual forces. Both forms of healing can be used as part of treatment for a range of emotional and physical illnesses.

**Structural integration:** A systematic approach to relieving patterns of stress and impaired functioning, structural integration seeks to correct misalignments in the body created by gravity and physical and psychological trauma. As in Rolfing, in ten sessions the practitioner uses hands, arms, and elbows to apply pressure to the fascia, or connective tissue, while the client participates through directed breathing.

**Tai chi/martial arts:** The martial arts are perhaps best known as means of self-defense, but they also are used to improve physical fitness and promote mental and spiritual development. The highly disciplined movements and forms are thought to unite body and mind and to bring balance to the individual's life. External methods (such as *karate* and *judo*) stress endurance and muscular strength, whereas internal methods (such as *tai chi* and *aikido*) stress relaxation and control. *Tai chi* has been used as part of treatment for back problems, ulcers, and stress.

**Therapeutic Touch:** Popularized by nursing professor Dolores Krieger, Therapeutic Touch is practiced by registered nurses and others to relieve pain and stress. The practitioner assesses where the person's energy field is weak or congested and then uses his or her hands to direct energy into the field to balance it.

**Trigger point/myotherapy:** Practitioners of this technique apply pressure to specific points on the body to relieve tension. Trigger points are tender, congested spots on muscle tissue that may radiate pain to other areas. Though the technique is similar to *shiatsu* or acupressure, this therapy uses Western anatomy and physiology as its basis.

**Yoga therapy:** This emerging field of practice uses yoga to address mental and physical problems while integrating body and mind. Practitioners work one-on-one or in group settings, assisting clients with yoga postures, sometimes combined with therapeutic verbal dialogue.

**Zero balancing:** This is a method for aligning body structure and body energy. Through touch akin to acupressure, the practitioner seeks to overcome imbalances in the structure/energetic interface of the body, which is said to exist beneath the level of conscious awareness. Zero balancing is often used for stress reduction.

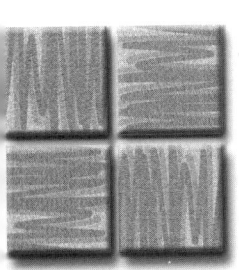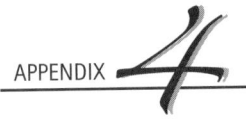

# Glossary of Computer and Internet Terms

**Bandwidth:** In a general sense, this term describes information-carrying capacity and can apply to telephone or network wiring as well as system buses, radio frequency signals, and monitors. Bandwidth is measured most accurately in cycles per second, or hertz (Hz), which is the difference between the lowest and highest frequencies transmitted. Bits or bytes per second are commonly used instead.

**Boolean operator:** The term for a number of conjunctions (AND, OR, NOT, and less commonly WITH or ADJ) used in constructing Boolean queries. More information on Boolean searching is available at the University of Albany library Web site <http://library.albany.edu/internet/boolean.html>.

**Browser:** In brief, a browser is the interface to the World Wide Web; it interprets hypertext links and lets one view sites and navigate from one Internet node to another. Among the companies that produce browsers are NCSA Mosaic, Netscape, and Microsoft and commercial services such as CompuServe, Prodigy, and America Online.

**CD-ROM (compact disc, read-only memory):** Used to store and play back computer data instead of digital audio. CD-ROMs can contain up to 650MB of data (though they often contain a lot less). CD-ROMs have become a favorite medium for installing programs because they cost only slightly more to manufacture than floppy disks and most major software applications come on at least five floppies.

**Cookie:** According to Netscape, cookies are a "general mechanism which server side connections can use to both store and retrieve information on the client side of the connection." In English, that means cookies are small data files written to the hard drive by some Web sites when one views them in the browser. These data files contain information the site can use to track things such as passwords, lists of pages one has visited, and the date when one last looked at a certain page.

**Crawler:** This term is practically synonymous with *spider*. However, since the advent of the WebCrawler site from AOL, moves are afoot to protect the word *crawler* as a trademark.

**Digital signature:** Forgery is a growing concern on the Internet. Digital signatures are a means of proving that a file or e-mail message belongs to a specific person, much as a driver's license proves identity. Digital signatures have the added benefit of verifying that one's message has not been tampered with. When one signs a message, a hash function, a computation that leaves a specific code, or digital fingerprint, is applied to the message. If the fingerprint on the recipient's message does not match the original fingerprint, the message has been altered. Digital signatures often are used with strong encryption software to create a secure channel of communication in which privacy and identity are protected.

**Domain name:** The domain name is at the right of the @ sign in an e-mail address, or about ten characters into a URL. The domain name of the Complementary Medicine Program Web site at the University of Maryland is **<http://www.compmed. umm.edu>**. Domain names have different extensions based on whether the domain belongs to a commercial enterprise (.com), and educational establishment (.edu), a government body (.gov), the military (.mil), a network (.net), or a nonprofit organization (.org).

**DVD:** Originally referred to as *digital video disks,* these high-capacity optical disks are now used to store everything from massive computer applications to full-length movies. Although similar in physical size and appearance to a compact disk or a CD-ROM, DVD is a huge leap from the 650MB of storage of its predecessor. A standard single-layer, single-sided DVD can store a whopping 4.7GB of data.

**File transfer protocol (FTP):** This Internet protocol is used to copy files between computers, usually a client and an archive site.

**Hard drive:** A hard drive is just a large disk that holds huge amounts of information, usually inside the case of a computer. Many persons often confuse the hard drive with the memory of the computer. Information remains on the hard drive even after the computer is turned off. When one saves a file, one saves it to the hard drive.

**Hypertext:** The term describes a nonsequential way of presenting information. Hypertext links information in a complex web of associations, powered by hyperlinks. Essentially a way of browsing information, hypertext is a way to describe how one learns information from a well-designed CD-ROM encyclopedia or from the World Wide Web.

**Information superhighway:** This buzzword from a speech by Al Gore refers to the plan by the Clinton/Gore administration to deregulate communication services and thus widen the scope of the Internet by opening carriers, such as television cable, to data communication. The term is widely and loosely used to mean the Internet.

**Internet:** The Internet originated in 1969, in the midst of the Cold War, as a nuke-proof communications network. As one might guess, the Internet received most of its early financing from the U.S. Department of Defense. Now, however, the Internet consists of countless networks and computers across the world that allow millions of persons to share information. The lines that carry most of the information are known as the *Internet backbone.* Although the government used to run the Internet, now major Internet service providers (ISPs) such as MCI, GTE, Sprint, UUNET, and ANS own portions of the backbone, which is good, because they have the motivation and the revenue to maintain the quality of these large networks.

**Internet protocol address (IP address):** This address is a unique string of numbers that identifies a computer on the Internet. These numbers usually are shown in groups separated by periods, like this: 123.123.23.2. All resources on the Internet must have an IP address or else they are not on the Internet at all.

**Java:** Sun Microsystems developed a programming language for adding animation and other action to Web sites. The small applications (called *applets*) that Java creates can play back on any graphical system that is Web-ready, but the Web browser has to be Java-capable for one to see it. According to a description by Sun, Java is a "simple, object-oriented, distributed, interpreted, robust, secure, architecture-neutral, portable, high-performance, multithreaded, dynamic, buzzword-compliant, general-purpose programming language." And Sun should know.

**JPEG (Joint Photographic Experts Group):** This file format for color-rich images was developed by the Joint Photographic Experts Group committee. JPEG compresses graphics of photographic color depth better than competing file formats such as GIF, and it retains a high degree of color fidelity. This makes JPEG files smaller and therefore quicker to download. One can choose how much to compress a JPEG file, but because the format is *lossy*, the smaller the file is compressed, the more color information will be lost. JPEG files can be viewed by a variety of downloadable software on the PC and Mac.

**Megabyte:** Although *mega* is Greek for a million, a megabyte actually contains 1,048,576 bytes (1024 × 1024 bytes). In other words, a million bytes is actually less than a megabyte. Remember that the next time you buy a hard disk or try to fit files onto a floppy disk. Abbreviated as MB.

**MHz (megahertz):** A *megahertz* is 1 million complete cycles per second. This unit is used most commonly to measure transmission speeds of electronic devices, such as the clock speed of a microprocessor, the small computer chip that handles data-related tasks.

**MPEG (Moving Pictures Experts Group):** MPEG is a standard for compressing sound and movie files into an attractive format for downloading, or even streaming, across the Internet. The MPEG-1 standard streams video and sound data at 150 kilobytes per second, the same rate as a single-speed CD-ROM drive, and manages the process by taking key frames of video and filling only the areas that change between the frames. Unfortunately, MPEG-1 produces only adequate quality video, far below that of standard TV.

**OS (operating system):** A computer by itself is essentially dumb bits of wire and silicon. An operating system knows how to talk to this hardware and can manage the functions of a computer, such as allocating memory, scheduling tasks, accessing disk drives, and supplying a user interface. Without an operating system, software developers would have to write programs that directly accessed hardware, essentially reinventing the wheel with every new program.

**Proxy server:** A proxy server is a system that caches items from other servers to speed up access. On the Web, a proxy first attempts to find data locally, and, if the data is not available, the server fetches it from the remote server where the data resides permanently.

**QuickTime:** Developed by Apple Computer, QuickTime is a method of storing sound, graphics, and movie files. A MOV file on the Web or on a CD-ROM is a QuickTime file. Although QuickTime was developed originally for the Macintosh, player software is now available for Windows and other platforms. If one does not have a QuickTime player, one can always download versions for a Mac or PC from the Apple Web site.

**RAM (random access memory):** When one runs an application like Microsoft Word, the program is called up from its permanent storage area (like the hard drive, floppy disk, or CD-ROM) and moved into the RAM, where it sends requests to the CPU. The computer should have as much RAM as is affordable so that it can work efficiently. Having lots of memory in a system for running operating systems such as Windows 2000 and XP and other advanced software applications is essential.

**Search engine:** When a user enters text into a search form, a program called a *search engine* analyzes the text and searches for matching terms in an index file, which was created using a search indexer. The search engine returns the results of its search using a results listing.

**Search form:** This HTML page lets users type in search terms and set various search options. For example, the main page on Google contains a search form. When a user enters a search, the search engine program compares the search criteria against an index file, which was created using a search indexer. The search engine returns the results of its search using a results listing.

**Search indexer:** This program analyzes documents such as Web pages and creates a searchable index file. The resulting index file is used by a search engine to locate files containing specific words or phrases.

**Spam (spiced ham):** Junk e-mail. Spam can be a mass mailing to bulletin boards, newsgroups, or lists of persons. Spam is usually not welcome.

**Spider:** Also known as a *Web spider*, this class of robot software explores the World Wide Web by retrieving a document and following all the hyperlinks in it. Web sites tend to be so well linked that a spider can cover vast amounts of the Internet by starting from just a few sites. After following the links, spiders generate catalogs that can be accessed by search engines. Popular search sites like Google, AltaVista, Excite, and Lycos use this method.

**Streaming:** Data is *streaming* when it is moving quickly from one piece of hardware to another and does not have to be all in one place for the destination device to do something with it. When the data on a hard disk is being written to a tape backup device, the date is streaming. When one watches a QuickTime movie on the Internet, the movie is not streaming because it must be downloaded fully before it can be played.

**T1:** T1 is a term coined by AT&T for a system that transfers digital signals at 1.544 megabits per second (as opposed to the ISDN standard of a mere 64 kilobits per second). Of course, if T1 does not cut it, T3 is available. (T2 seems to have been bypassed altogether.)

**TCP/IP (transmission control protocol/Internet protocol):** These two protocols were developed by the U.S. military to allow computers to talk to each other over long distance networks. IP is responsible for moving packets of data between nodes. TCP is responsible for verifying delivery from client to server. TCP/IP forms the basis of the Internet and is built into every common modern operating system (including all versions of Unix, the Mac OS, and the latest versions of Windows).

**World Wide Web:** Also known as the WWW, the W3, or most often simply as the Web, the World Wide Web originally was developed by CERN labs in Geneva,

Switzerland. Continuing development of the Web is overseen by the World Wide Web Consortium. The Web can be described as a client/server hypertext system for retrieving information across the Internet. On the Web, everything is represented as hypertext (in HTML format) and is linked to other documents by their URLs. The Web encompasses its native HTTP protocol, as well as FTP, Gopher, and Telnet.

**Uniform resource locator:** URLs are the Internet equivalent of addresses. How do they work? Like other types of addresses, they move from the general to the specific (from ZIP code to recipient, so to speak). The following URL, for example, **<http://www.nccam.nih.gov/htdig/search.html>** first indicates the protocol (*http://*), then the server address or domain (*www.nccam.nih.gov*), and then the directory (*/htdig/search*).

**ZIP:** An open standard for compression and decompression used widely for PC download archives, ZIP was developed by Phil Katz for his DOS-based program PKZip, and is now used widely on Windows-based programs such as WinZip and Drag and Zip. The file extension given to ZIP files is .zip.

# Index

## A

Achoo, 23
ACUBASE, 34t
  access and URL, 110t
ACULARS, access by e-mail, 110t
Acupuncture, 5, 54-60, 56f, 57t
  books on, 58-59
  Cochrane Systematic Reviews of, 125t
  FDA reclassification process for, 54
  Internet resources on, 55, 56f, 57t, 58
  journals on, 59-60
  NIH consensus statement on, 54, 55f
  professional organizations for, 60
  special online reports and articles
    about, 86-87
Addictions, NCCAM-funded research
  on, 93t
Adverse effects, information sources on,
  28-29
Aging, NCCAM-funded research on, 93t
AGRICOLA, access and URL, 110t
AGRICultural OnLine Access, 34t
  access and URL, 110t
Alexander technique, Cochrane
  Systematic Reviews of, 125t
Allied and Complementary Medicine, 34t
  access and URL, 110t
AltaVista, 23
Alternative Medicine Foundation, 96
AltHealthWatch, 34t
  access and URL, 110t

AMED, access and URL, 110t
American Accreditation HealthCare
  Commission, URL, audience,
  mechanism, philosophy, 49t
American Dietetic Association, position
  papers from, 73
American Medical Association, URL,
  audience, mechanism,
  philosophy, 49t
American WholeHealth, resources of,
  100
Andreesen, Marc, 3-4
Arthritis, NCCAM-funded research on,
  93t
Asian medicine, 5
Ask Dr. Weil, 1, 127
Asthma, evidence-based summaries
  on, 57t
Atkins diet, 6
Ayurveda, components of, 5

## B

Back pain, evidence-based summaries
  on, 57t
Bandolier, 30, 31t, 96
  consumer health information of, 124
  evidence-based summaries of, 107t
    on acupuncture, 55, 56f
    on diet therapies, 71, 72t-73t
    on herbal medicine, 60, 61t-63t
    on homeopathy, 77, 79t

Bandolier *(Continued)*
    on manual therapies, 67, 68t
    on mind-body therapies, 75-77
    on spiritual healing, 80, 81t
BioMed
    acupuncture resources of, 55
    homeopathy in, 78
Body-based therapies, 6
Boolean operators, 20-21
Botanicals, NCCAM-funded research
    on, 93t
*British Medical Journal*
    acupuncture resources of, 55
    diet therapy resources in, 71
    herbal medicine resources of, 60
    homeopathy in, 77-78
    manual therapy resources of, 67

C

CAM. *See* Complementary and
    alternative medicine
CAMline, access and URL, 111t
Canada, Internet resources from, 124
Canadian Natural Health Products
    Directorate
    consumer health resources of, 122
    web site of, 91
Cancer, NCCAM-funded research on,
    93t-94t
Cancer Information Service, 87, 89
Cancer Trials Database, 121
Cancer Trials web site, 87, 89
Cardiovascular disease, NCCAM-funded
    research on, 94t
Case sensitive searches, 20
Centers for Disease Control and
    Prevention (CDC)
    consumer health resources of, 122
    web site of, 90-91
CHIROLARS. *See* Manual, Alternative
    and Natural Therapy Database
Chiropractic
    books on, 68-69
    Internet resources on, 67-68, 70

Chiropractic *(Continued)*
    journals on, 69
    NCCAM-funded research on, 94t
CISCOM, 31t
    evidence-based resources of, 107t
Clinical trials, Internet resources on,
    91, 92t
ClinicalTrials.gov, 34t
    access and URL, 111t
    consumer health information on, 123
Cochrane Collaboration Complementary
    Medicine Field, 95, 143-160
    abstracts of, on diet therapies, 71
    CAM protocols of, 153t-156t
    CAM reviews of, 145t-152t
    completed reviews of, 159-160
    history of, 143-144
    library of, 144
    medical subject headings in, 158-159
    mission of, 143
    review registry of, 158
    spiritual healing resources of, 80
    structure of, 144, 160
    trial registry of, 158
Cochrane Collaboration Consumer
    Network, 95, 96f
Cochrane Complementary Medicine
    Field, 31t, 157-158
    evidence-based resources of, 107t
Cochrane Consumer Network, consumer
    reviews of, 124, 125t-126t
Cochrane Library, 30, 32t
    acupuncture resources of, 67
    acupuncture web site of, 55, 56f
    evidence-based resources of, 108t
    herbal medicine abstracts in, 60
    resources of, 99
    searching, 42-44
Cochrane Systematic Reviews for
    Consumers, summaries of,
    125t-126t
Combined Health Information
    Database, 87
    consumer health resources of, 120

Complementary and alternative
    medicine. *See also* specific types
  associations for, 128t
  classification of, 5b
  conditions treated by, 9t
  consensus statements on, 84
  databases for research in, 110t-115t
  defined, 4
  directories for, 124, 127
  evidence-based resources in,
    107t-109t. *See also* Bandolier,
    evidence-based summaries of
  expenditures for, 8t
  glossary of terms, 167-172
  lack of professional standards in,
    137-138
  limits of scientific knowledge about,
    138
  literature review for, 30
  newsletters on, 105-106, 106t
  physician use of and interest in, 84
  professional books on, 100-102
  professional journals on, 103-105
  reasons for using, 9-10
  special online reports and articles
    about, 84-87
  technology and uses for generating
    information on, 140t
  types used, 10, 10t
  use of, by country, 53
  users of, 7-9, 8t
Complementary and alternative
    medicine web sites
  evaluating, 48, 50-51
  use of, 1-2
Computer Decency Act of 1996, 46
Computer terms, glossary of, 173-177
Confidentiality, protection of, 133
Consent, informed, 131-132
ConsumerLab.com, resources of, 100
Consumers
  health information for, 117-130
  Internet use by, 117-118
  quality and safety issues of, 121-122
  resources for, 122-129
  types of/conditions of, 118-121

Continuing medical education in CAM,
    organizations offering, 161-166
Contraindications, information sources
    on, 28-29
Craniofacial disorders, NCCAM-funded
    research on, 94t
Cumulative Index to Nursing and
    Allied Health, 34t
  access and URL, 111t

**D**

Databases, 30, 31t-33t, 34t-39t
  research, 110t-115t
Datadiwan, 35t
  access and URL, 111t
Dietary supplements, government web
    site on, 90
Dietary supplements/food labeling
    electronic newsletter, 90
Diet/nutritional therapies, 6, 71-75
  Bandolier evidence-based summaries
    of, 71, 72t
  books on, 73-74
  Internet resources on, 71, 74-75
  professional organizations for practi-
    tioners of, 74
Directory search tools, 17
Dr. Duke's Phytochemical and
    Ethnobotanical Databases, 35t
  access and URL, 111t

**E**

Education, continuing medical,
    organizations offering, 161-166
Efficacy, information sources on, 28
eHealth Code of Ethics, URL, audience,
    mechanism, philosophy, 49t
EMBASE, 35t
  access and URL, 111t
Energy therapies, 6-7
Ethical issues. *See* Legal/ethical issues
EthnobotDB, 35t
  access and URL, 112t
Excite, 24

**F**

Federal Trade Commission
    consumer health resources of, 122
    web site of, 91
Fellowships, CAM, 164-165
Fibromyalgia, evidence-based
    summaries on, 57t
Fields, 21
FirstGov, 89-90
Food and Drug Administration, 46-47
    acupuncture reclassification process
        for, 54
    consumer health resources of, 121-122
    web site of, 47f, 90
FTC. *See* U.S. Federal Trade Commission

**G**

Google, 24
Google search, 16, 16f
Government resources
    for consumers, 118-121
    for professionals and researchers, 87-90

**H**

Headache, evidence-based summaries
    on, 57t
Health and safety claims, tracking of,
    45-46
Health care, information generated on,
    15-16
Health Improvement Institute, URL,
    audience, mechanism, philosophy,
    49t
Health on the Net, URL, audience,
    mechanism, philosophy, 49t
Health professionals
    CAM resources for, 83-116
    products and sites for, 98-105,
        106t-115t
Health Protection Branch, Canada
    consumer health resources of, 122
    web site of, 91
Health sites
    number of, 16
    quality initiatives for rating, 47-48

Healthfinder, consumer health
    information on, 124
Healthnotes, resources of, 99
Healthwell, 124
Herbal medicine, 5, 60-67
    Bandolier evidence-based summaries
        on, 61t-63t
    books on, 65
    Internet resources on, 60, 64, 66-67
    journals on, 65-66
    professional organizations for, 66
    special online reports and articles
        about, 86
Herbal therapies, 6
    Cochrane Systematic Reviews of,
        125t-126t
HerbMed, 32t, 35t
    access and URL, 112t
    evidence-based resources of, 108t
Hi-Ethics, URL, audience, mechanism,
    philosophy, 49t
Homeopathy, 77-80
    Bandolier evidence-based summaries
        on, 77, 79t
    Cochrane Systematic Reviews of, 126t
    principles of, 5
    special online reports and articles
        about, 86
Hom-Inform Database, 35t
    access and URL, 112t
HTML, 3
HTTP, 3

**I**

Informed consent, 131-132
Integrative medicine, trends in, 7
Integrative Medicine Communications,
    resources of, 99-100
InteliHealth, 127
International Bibliographic Information
    on Dietary Supplements, 36t
    access and URL, 112t
Internet
    challenges pertaining to, 137-138
    evaluating CAM resources of, 45-52

Internet *(Continued)*
  evaluating information on, 16
  future of, 136-139
  glossary of terms, 173-177
  history of, 2-4
  influence of, 1
  medical information on, 10
  number of users of, 4
  quality of information on, 138
  reasons for using, 10, 11t, 12t
  searching, 15-26
    defining question in, 17
    structured approach to, 16-19
    tools/methods for, 17-18
  users of, 11-12

J

Journals
  acupuncture, 59-60
  chiropractic, 69
  herbal medicine, 65-66
  homeopathy, 78-79
  mind-body medicine, 77

K

Keyword searches, 17-18

L

Legal/ethical issues, 131-135
  informed consent, 131-132
  licensing/record keeping, 134
  physician/patient and provider/
    patient relationships, 132
  privacy and security, 133
  web sites on, 132-133
Licensing, of online communications,
  134

M

Manipulative therapies, 6
MANTIS, access and URL, 112t
Manual, Alternative and Natural
  Therapy Database, 36t
  access and URL, 112t

Manual therapies, 67-70. *See also*
  Chiropractic; Massage; Osteopathy
  Bandolier evidence-based summaries
    of, 67, 68t
Massage
  Bandolier evidence-based summaries
    on, 68t
  books on, 69
  Internet resources on, 70
McMaster University Alternative
  Medicine Resources, 124
MD Consult, 30
  resources of, 99
MedCertain, URL, audience,
  mechanism, philosophy, 49t
Medical literature, getting overview
  of, 30
Medical schools, CAM continuing
  education in, 161-163
Medical system, alternative, 5
Medicinal Plants of Native America
  Database, 36t
  access and URL, 113t
Medicine, Asian, 5
MEDLINE/PubMed, access and URL,
  113t
MEDLINE, 30
MEDLINEplus, consumer health
  information on, 123-124
MEDLINE/PubMed, 36t
  access and URL, 113t
MedWebPlus: Alternative Medicine, 127
Metasearches, 18
MICROMEDEX Complementary &
  Alternative Medicine Series, 37t
  access and URL, 113t
MICROMEDEX Herbal & Alternative
  Remedies, 37t
  access and URL, 113t
Mind-body therapies, 6, 75-77
  Bandolier evidence-based summaries
    of, 76t
  books on, 75-76
  Internet resources for, 75

Mind-body therapies *(Continued)*
  journals on, 77
  professional organizations for
    practitioners of, 77
Minus signs, 19

**N**

National Cancer Institute
  CAM on web site of, 87, 88f
  consumer health resources of, 120-121
National Center for Biotechnology
    Information, databases of, 40. *See
    also* MEDLINE; PubMed
National Center for Complementary
    and Alternative Medicine, 37t, 87
  clinical trials recruiting volunteers,
    92t
  clinical trials research funded by, 122
  consumer health resources of, 118-119
  Public Information Clearinghouse of,
    119
  research centers funded by, 93t-95t
  web site for, 54
National Institutes of Health
  consensus statement on acupuncture,
    54, 55f
  National Center for Complementary
    and Alternative Medicine web
    site of, 1
  number of people using, 13
  Office of Dietary Supplements of, 90
Native American Ethnobotany
    Database, 37t
  access and URL, 113t
Natural Medical Protocols for Doctors,
    37t
  access and URL, 114t
Natural Medicines Comprehensive
    Database, 38t
  access and URL, 114t
  resources of, 100
Natural Products ALERT, 38t
  access and URL, 114t
Naturopathy, principles of, 5

Nausea, postsurgical, evidence-based
    summaries on, 57t
NCCAM. *See* National Center for Com-
    plementary and Alternative Medicine
Nesting, 21
Neurodegenerative disease, NCCAM-
    funded research on, 94t
Neurological disorders, NCCAM-
    funded research on, 94t
Newsletters
  for CAM professionals, 105-106, 106t
  on consumer health, 129
Northern Light, 24
Nurses. *See* Health professionals
Nutritional therapies. *See*
    Diet/nutritional therapies
Nutritionals Adverse Event Monitoring
    System, 38t
  access and URL, 114t

**O**

Office of Alternative Medicine. *See*
    National Center for
    Complementary and Alternative
    Medicine
Office of Dietary Supplements,
    National Institutes of Health, 90
OMNI. *See* Organising Medical
    Networked Information
Operation Cure All, 45
Organising Medical Networked
    Information, 96
  consumer health information of, 124
  URL, audience, mechanism,
    philosophy, 49t
Ornish diet, 6
Orthomolecular therapies, 6
Osteoarthritis, evidence-based
    summaries on, 57t
Osteopathy, Internet resources on, 67
Ovid, searching, 44
Ovid Best Evidence Collection, 32t
  evidence-based resources of, 108t
Ovid Online Digital Collection, 30

## P

Parentheses, 21
Patent Database, 38t
  access and URL, 114t
PC-SPES, 138
Pediatrics, NCCAM-funded research on, 95t
Phrases, searching for, 20
Physician-patient relationship, legal/ethical issues in, 132
Physicians. *See* Health professionals
PhytoNet, 39t
  access and URL, 114t
Phytotherapies.org Monograph Database, 39t
  access and URL, 115t
Plus signs, 19
POEMs (Patient Oriented Evidence That Matters), 32t, 108t
Poisonous Plant Database, 39t
  access and URL, 115t
Prayer, 80, 81t
  Cochrane Systematic Reviews of, 126t
Privacy, ethical issues in, 133
Professional organizations, 128t
  for acupuncture, 60
  for diet therapy practitioners, 74
  for herbal medicine practitioners, 66
  for homeopathy, 79-80
  for manual therapy professionals, 69
  for spiritual healing practitioners, 81-82
Professional training, 165-166
Provider-patient relationship, legal/ethical issues in, 132
PsychInfo, 39t
  access and URL, 115t
PubMed, 30
  access and URL, 110t
  CAM on, 31t, 87, 107t, 110t
  consumer health resources of, 120
  evidence-based resources of, 107t
  searching, 40-42

## Q

*Qi*, 5
*Qi gong*, 5, 6-7
Quality, 45-47
  awards for, 49t
  government web sites on, 90-91
  information sources on, 29
Quality initiatives, 47-48
Queries, composing, 21-22
Questions, defining, 17

## R

*Reiki*, 6-7
  Internet resources on, 82
Research
  databases for, 110t-115t
  Internet resources on, 91
  news sites on, 105
Research organizations, 96-98
  NCCAM-funded, 93t-95t
Residency training, 164-165

## S

Safety issues
  government web sites on, 90-91
  information sources on, 28-29
St. John's wort as AIDS treatment, 46
Search engine tools, 17-18
  preferred, 19b
Search engines
  directory with, 18
  specific, 22-24
Search tools, 15
  multiengine, 18
Searches
  for CAM, 27-44
    databases for, 34t-39t
    specific resources for, 30, 31t-33t
    and story of fisherman and net, 33
    strategies for, 27-30
    timeliness and, 28
  conducting and refining, 19-25
    advanced methods, 20-21
    simple methods, 19-20

Searches *(Continued)*
  interpreting results of, 25-26
  problems and remedies for, 22
Security, ethical issues in, 133
Servers, 15
Smoking cessation, evidence-based
    summaries on, 57t
Spiritual healing, 80-82
Stemming, 19-20
Subject searches, 17
SUMSearch, 32t
  evidence-based resources of, 109t

**T**

Tai chi, Cochrane Systematic Reviews
    of, 126t
Temporomandibular joint dysfunction,
    evidence-based summaries on, 57t
Therapeutic Touch, 6
  Bandolier evidence-based summaries
      of, 81t
  Internet resources on, 82
TRIP Database, 33t
  evidence-based resources of, 109t

**U**

Uniform resource locators (URLs), 15
U.S. Federal Trade Commission,
    Operation Cure All of, 46, 46f
United Kingdom, Internet resources
    from, 124
University of Maryland Complementary
    Medicine Program Databases, 33t,
    109t

URLs, 15
UseNet, 3

**V**

Vomiting, postsurgical, evidence-based
    summaries on, 57t

**W**

Web. *See* Internet; World wide web
Web browser, origins of, 3
Web sites, evaluating, guidelines for, 48,
    50-51
WebMD/Medscape, 127
  resources of, 99
Weil, Andrew, 1, 127
White House Commission on
    Complementary and Alternative
    Medicine Policy, 89, 89f
  consumer health information on, 124
WholeHealthMD, 127
Women's health, NCCAM-funded
    research on, 93t
World Health Organization, consumer
    health resources of, 122
World wide web. *See also* Internet
  documents contained in, 15
  history of, 2-4
  origins of, 2-3

**Y**

Yahoo, 25
Yoga, Cochrane Systematic Reviews of,
    126t